SDI and the
ALTERNATIVES

SDI and the
ALTERNATIVES

SIMON P. WORDEN

1991

National Defense University Press
Fort Lesley J. McNair
Washington, DC 20319–6000

National Defense University Press Publications

To increase general knowledge and inform discussion, NDU Press publishes books on subjects relating to US national security.

Each year, in this effort, the National Defense University, through the Institute for National Strategic Studies, hosts about two dozen Senior Fellows who engage in original research on national security issues. NDU Press publishes the best of this research.

In addition, the Press publishes other especially timely or distinguished writing on national security, as well as new editions of out-of-print defense classics, and books based on University-sponsored conferences concerning national security affairs.

Proofread under contract by Azonic Services Corporation, Potomac, Maryland. Indexed under contract by Shirley Kessel, Primary Sources Research, Chevy Chase, Maryland.

NDU Press publications are sold by the US Government Printing Office. For ordering information, call (202) 783-3238 or write to: Superintendent of Documents, US Government Printing Office, Washington, DC 20402.

First printing, July 1991

Library of Congress Cataloging-in-Publication Data
Worden, Simon P.
    SDI and alternatives / Simon P. Worden.
      p.   cm.
    Includes bibliographical references and index.
    1. Strategic Defense Initiative. 2. United States—Military policy. 3. Deterrence (Strategy) 4. Nuclear warfare. 5. Disarmament. I. Title.
UG743.W67   1991
358.1'74—dc20   # 22623250   90–20579
                                  CIP

CONTENTS

Figures

FOREWORD

The controversial, sometimes emotional national debate over strategic defense has been overshadowed recently by other, even weightier national and global issues. Research programs for the Strategic Defense Initiative continue, however, and the debate is likely to resume as visible results of that research begin to compete for a share of the nation's budget. It is in the national interest that this debate proceed in an atmosphere of rational, objective analysis.

This study—by an experienced scientist and military expert—provides a basis for such analysis. Colonel Simon P. Worden, US Air Force, considers strategic defense in the context of four competing strategic theories: (1) deterrence through mutual assured destruction, (2) deterrence through nuclear warfighting, (3) deterrence relying on non-nuclear defense, and (4) disarmament. He points out misconceptions and exaggerations of earlier SDI debate, taking to task those in the scientific community who abandoned objective analysis to pursue a political agenda. His fundamental theme is that non-nuclear, space-based defense is not only feasible, but in some ways preferable to reliance on weapons of mass destruction. To support his case, he outlines the phases of a proposed actual system.

As Worden notes, the ultimate decisions on strategic defense are up to the American people and their representatives. Such decisions will no doubt take in a range of factors—economic, political, technical, and ethical—as all important national decisions should. Worden offers a reasoned case for strategic defense as an alternative strategy for deterring war.

J.A. BALDWIN
Vice Admiral, US Navy
President, National Defense
University

SDI and the
ALTERNATIVES

INTRODUCTION: THE ELEMENTS IN THE STRATEGIC DEBATE

As the sun rose over Sierra Blanca Mountain on the morning of July 16, 1945, it was momentarily matched by the brilliance of the world's first atomic explosion, at the United States' New Mexico Trinity site. This ushered in a new era in military thought—or so the bomb's inventors believed. Out of the mass destruction potential of nuclear weapons, the intellectual community believed it had the way to end war—one of mankind's oldest hopes. The theory of how nuclear weapons can end war is now known as Mutual Assured Destruction, or MAD.

Most Americans believe MAD is the basis of US nuclear strategy. I will show in the following chapters that it is not. Rather than ending all thoughts of war, nuclear weapons have been integrated into a "warfighting" strategy. In this complicated plan, nuclear weapons, along with non-nuclear weapons, prevent war because we are able to fight and prevail if the need arises.

Four Paths to Peace

Technology has marched ahead since 1945. We have entered a new era—the space age. Military thought has only begun to incorporate space. The Soviet Union has, quite correctly, identified space as equal to nuclear weapons in its impact on military affairs.

MAD, nuclear warfighting, and space have driven the United States into an intense, emotional strategic debate. Strategists have hardened their positions and narrowed their minds to such a degree that the debate has come to resemble a medieval clash of true believers—religious zealotry replacing reason. President Reagan's introduction of a new strategy based in large

1

part on emerging space technologies—the Strategic Defense Initiative, or SDI—has driven the debate to new levels of irrationality. In this book, I hope to consider SDI in a national context with respect to its competing strategic theories.

Three of the four strategic concepts in the United States are "deterrent"—the other is anti-deterrent. In order to understand these approaches, one must first understand two basic concepts—*deterrence* and *damage limitation.*

Deterrence comprises the actions, forces, and strategies a nation takes to prevent war. The three US deterrent theories are:

1. Mutual Assured Destruction (MAD) or vulnerability-based deterrence.

2. Flexible Response or nuclear warfighting deterrence.

3. Defense-reliant deterrence or non-nuclear deterrence.

There is a fourth concept—one that rejects deterrence as unnecessary. This strategy regards the adversarial relationship which deterrence perpetuates as the potential source of war. I identify this approach as:

4. Total Disarmament.

Damage Limitation comprises what to do if deterrence fails. Damage limitation must be separated from deterrence. There are at least four damage limitation possibilities.

1. Civil Defense.

2. Preemptive strikes—attack their forces before they destroy yours.

3. Active strategic defense.

4. Hope—if you believe there is nothing we can do if nuclear war starts.

Each strategy's adherents have radically different views on damage limitation. MAD and disarmament advocates regard damage limitation alternative four, hope, as the only possibility. Indeed, these strategists believe that other damage limitation approaches actually weaken deterrence.

One other point to keep in mind is my use of the term "strategists" to describe adherents to some approaches. The adherents of MAD, in particular, claim that it isn't a strategy—but a fact of life.[1] This is misleading, for as I will show later there are volumes of strategic analysis and arguments defending MAD over other strategies. MAD is as much a strategy as any other.

I find that a four-parameter framework allows me to quickly identify the differences in each approach. Figure 1 illustrates the four strategic theories in that framework.

The first parameter is the role of offensive forces. Most of the debate over strategic concepts in the 1980s focused on this strategic element. For example, the adherents of each strategy have been either wildly enthusiastic, or appalled, respectively, over the deployment of the MX and Midgetman ICBMs. Those who like the latter system tend to hate the former. These opinions have very little to do with the technological features of the two but have everything to do with strategy.

The second element is the role of damage-limiting capabilities—specifically civil defense and active defense. Some strategists reject these altogether, others argue that they enhance deterrence.

Arms control is the third element of national security strategy that has come to take center stage in the public eye. The view that arms control can enhance security is controversial. It assumes that our adversary can be induced to take actions to better US security. Whether this is a sensible approach or not, arms control goals are radically different depending on the strategy arms control is intended to support.

The last element is not so much a strategic input as a measure of the strategist's state of mind—who or what is the enemy? To most Americans—unfortunately stereotyped by US intellectuals as "Joe Average" and his wife "Harriet Housewife"—the answer is obvious. The enemy is the godless "commies" in Moscow. However, the strategic theorists often have a much different answer. Ironically, the "enemy" to some strategists is in Washington, DC, not Moscow.

Vulnerability-Based Nuclear Deterrence

The basic dogma of Mutual Assured Destruction (MAD), also known as vulnerability-based nuclear deterrence, is simple.

	VULNERABILITY-BASED	NUCLEAR WAR FIGHTING	NON-NUCLEAR	DISARMAMENT
ROLE OF OFFENSE	DESTROY SOVIET SOCIETY (1000 WARHEADS) ✓	DESTROY SOVIET MILITARY FORCES IN 2nd STRIKE ✓✓	DEFEAT CONVENTIONAL FORCES ✓	NONE ✗
ROLE OF DEFENSE	NONE (UNLESS PERFECT) ✗	PROTECT RETALIATORY FORCES ✓	DEFEAT SOVIET STRATEGIC ROCKET TROOPS ✓✓	NONE ✗
ROLE OF ARMS CONTROL	PERSUADE SOVIETS TO MAKE THEMSELVES VULNERABLE ✓✓	REDUCE SOVIET FIRST-STRIKE FORCES ✓	PERSUADE SOVIETS TO ADOPT A DEFENSIVE STRATEGY ✓	PERSUADE SOVIETS U.S. IS NOT A THREAT ✓✓
WHO'S THE ENEMY	INSTABILITY (U.S. GOVERNMENT SOMETIMES)	SOVIET STRATEGIC ROCKET TROOPS (FIRST STRIKE)	SOVIET WAR PLANS	U.S. MILITARISM & SOVIET MILITARISM

Figure 1. The Four Strategic Theories. Each approach features radically different roles for offensive forces, defensive forces, and arms control. Most telling is the identity of the "enemy" in each strategy.

That simplicity is its strength. If a weapon is so terrible that using it would end civilization, the very existence of such a weapon should end war. For if any conflict risks the end of the world, no one in his right mind would enter such a conflict. MAD adherents hold that nuclear bombs are such weapons. Thus, perpetual peace is assured when rational nations possess the minimum number of weapons needed to end the world. MAD's basic tenets emerged from the scientific and intellectual communities soon after World War II. The seminal work was Bernard Brodie's appropriately titled book, *The Absolute Weapon*.[2] MAD's simplicity has caught the imagination of most of the so-called ''intellectual'' community, particularly those physicists who invented nuclear weapons.

Offensive nuclear weapons are the mainstay of MAD military forces. Yet MAD strategists insist that these weapons must be kept to the absolute minimum number necessary to destroy the world. To keep this number as small as possible, MAD adherents turn not to technology, but to politics. Their goal is to maximize the destructiveness of nuclear weapons in the minds of the public and decisionmakers. In the 1960s MAD was briefly our declared strategy, albeit not actual US policy. Calculations from that era suggested that roughly 1000 megatons would assure destruction—destroying 25 percent of a nation's population and 50 percent of its industry. In recent years, MAD strategists have progressively lowered these requirements to about 10 percent population destruction. Moreover, certain physicists have advanced reasons—especially the so-called ''nuclear winter''—for lowering the end-of-the-world threshold to about 100 megatons.

Defensive forces and efforts are anathema to MAD. The very suggestion that damage can be limited runs counter to MAD's end-of-the-world requirement. MAD theorists fear that a public believing that defense is possible is a public which has rejected the premise that nuclear war is unthinkable. On a less dogmatic plane, defenses add uncertainty and make it more difficult to calculate the minimum necessary weapons to assure destruction. This uncertainty, they argue, will drive an offense-defense arms race. Of course, MAD advocates have no objection to perfect defense which can *replace* deterrence. We must remember, though, that it is MAD deterrence they are talking about.

The primary MAD tool is arms control. It is far more important than details of offensive or defensive forces. For MAD to work, both sides must accept its premises. Arms control's primary goal is getting the other side to accept MAD. First, the other side must be persuaded to make themselves vulnerable—that is, defenseless. This isn't easy with a defense-minded nation such as the Soviet Union. Second, arms control must get agreements with the MAD partner to reduce offensive weapons to the minimum level.

Who is MAD's enemy? It is not the Soviet Union—which, after all, must cooperate and become our arms control partner. Instead, MAD fears something called "instability." This is any move, often one taken by the US Government, which does not move closer to MAD. In recent years two moves have been particularly "destabilizing": First, moves by the nuclear warfighters to acquire new warfighting weapons, such as MX. Second, and viewed in a more sinister light, are efforts by the third deterrent school, the defenders, to show that nuclear weapons can be defended against (namely, through SDI) or survived (through civil defense).

Retaliation-Based Nuclear Deterrence

While academics debated MAD's philosophical niceties, more down-to-earth strategists became alarmed over growing Soviet military power. MAD did not seem to deter Soviet adventurism; indeed the side less afraid of nuclear war had an advantage. The nuclear warfighters believe that the only way to deter an aggressor is to be able to fight and win, or at least deny victory to the opponent, at all levels of conflict. Winning, of course, must be in terms of values recognized by the aggressor. In the 1940s and 1950s, this policy was simple nuclear "massive retaliation." With growing Soviet power in the 1960s and beyond, a more encompassing approach, "flexible response," emerged. The goal was, and still is today, to show to the Soviets that we can defeat their aggression at whatever level of conflict they initiate—and that we can win at higher levels of conflict as well, so-called "escalation dominance." Nuclear warfighting has always been, and remains today, US deterrent strategy.

Nuclear offensive forces are the dominant, if not the sole element of nuclear warfighting deterrence. Our nuclear forces must be sufficiently numerous to survive an enemy initial or "first" strike and to retaliate against the enemy's military forces. The retaliation must be strong to destroy those enemy military forces as an effective fighting instrument. In addition, the nuclear warfighters accept one MAD premise inasmuch as they seek to maintain a final reserve sufficient to destroy Soviet society. Survivable and accurate nuclear forces are the key to warfighting strategies. To ensure destruction of the thousands of Soviet military targets, we need thousands of warheads. Most Soviet military targets are small military units or facilities—targets which may be structurally reinforced (hardened) and also defended. To destroy these targets, giant city-killing bombs are almost useless—we need small, accurate nuclear weapons, and the trend has been toward smaller, more accurate nuclear weapons. The current US arsenal has only one quarter of its 1960s megatonnage. Since the number of enemy military targets is in the many thousands—our arsenal has grown to about 10,000 warheads, far larger and more capable than the MAD alternative.

Since our deterrent forces must be able to fight and prevail, this strategy has an implicit assumption that nuclear war is possible. For this reason, strategic defenses are accepted, but generally not given very high priority. Nuclear warfighting's architect is none other than the classic military strategist, Karl von Clausewitz. The traditional Clausewitz approach regards offensive forces as the tools of victory—but uses defensive capability as a valuable complement. Until the situation is right for a crushing offensive blow, defensive forces must protect these offensive forces and capabilities. Moreover, since nuclear war is not unthinkable—albeit totally unacceptable—damage-limiting means such as civil defense are valuable. These defensive capabilities are accepted and encouraged by nuclear warfighters—provided they do not detract from the offensive forces.

Arms control takes the back seat in nuclear warfighting deterrence. It contributes only if it can induce the enemy to make it easier and cheaper for us to defeat his military forces.

The Soviets also have a nuclear warfighting strategy. Thus it is hard to imagine their agreeing to offensive reductions which would make it easier for us to beat them. It is possible that arms control can preserve a precarious balance where neither side is sure of victory—and preserve it at lower overall force levels. But if the United States and Soviet Union view a particular weapon system differently—that is, we think the Soviet SS-18 ICBM is more potent than they do—it would be impossible to arrive at an agreed reduction that both sides find equitable. Arms control prospects under this strategy, as the decades of experience have shown, are bleak.

The nuclear warfighter's enemy is the Soviet Union. But the Soviets are not unqualifiedly the greatest evil. The nuclear warfighter still places not having a war above all else. It is a specific Soviet action—the first strike—which is feared. Soviet strategy is also nuclear warfighting, but with the assumption that the Soviets will preempt. Slightly different from a first strike, a "bolt from the blue" occurs without any prior crisis or warning. The Soviets would only strike first, however, if they thought a Western attack were imminent. The nuclear warfighter's enemy is the Soviet preemptive strike which could wipe out our ability to retaliate effectively against the Soviet military.

Non-Nuclear Deterrence

Every US President since Harry Truman has stated a goal of not only deterring nuclear war, but getting rid of nuclear weapons as well. However, as long as nuclear weapons are the basis of deterrence, as they are with MAD and nuclear warfighting, these two goals will remain mutually exclusive. Non-nuclear deterrence, relying principally on defensive capabilities, is a way to resolve this dilemma.

Non-nuclear deterrence seeks to deny all elements of Soviet strategic power and strategy with non-nuclear means. Its end objective is to drive the Soviets themselves into accepting a non-nuclear, non-offensive strategy. The tools for the former objective are technical, but the latter goal is an arms control one. The SDI is this effort's centerpiece. It addresses what US strategists feel is the central element of the Soviets' offensive nuclear strategy—their strategic nuclear forces. As I show later, this view is not wholly correct. Soviet conventional ground forces are regaining their traditional role as the mainstay of Soviet military power.

The principal US tool for moving to this new strategy is space. The United States has always had maximum leverage when it can introduce new elements into the strategic equation—in the 1990s and beyond, that new element will be space. Whenever the currency of military power is at the cutting edge of technology, as it is with space technology, the United States has an advantage.

Starting in reverse order of strategic elements, this strategy seeks to deny Soviet strategy. In this case the "enemy" is not instability, or even the Soviet first strike—it is simply the overall Soviet war plan. The idea here is not new. The basis of a 2400-year-old strategy, first written by the Chinese General Sun Tzu, was to deny enemy war plans, thus avoiding engaging him on the battlefield.[3] But what is Soviet strategy? Fortunately, the Soviets take a very mathematical view of military matters—quantifying what it takes to win in a "Correlation of Forces (COF)" analysis.

During the 1960s the Soviets developed detailed quantitative COF equations for nuclear war.[4] Their objective was to build their nuclear forces to a level where the nuclear COF would be greatly in their favor, should they find themselves in a war. Their COF includes comparisons of total nuclear striking power (megatonnage), vulnerability to enemy first strikes, and effectiveness of the opposing sides' defenses. By the 1990s the Soviet Union had built a formidable COF advantage over the United States.[5]

To deny the Soviet COF, we must develop non-nuclear defenses good enough to wipe out the advantage they have built up, and assure that they cannot recover this advantage in the future. This is the goal of the SDI—to show that such defenses are feasible and to prepare to deploy them. Effective defenses are thus a primary element of this strategy.

Soviet nuclear offensive forces are only one pillar of Soviet military strategy. We must also deny the other fundamental pillar of their strategy—their conventional forces. Conventional

COF relations are more difficult to calculate than the nuclear COF. However, Soviet conventional strategy has been well documented and has remained the same for the past century. The goal is to prepare locally overwhelming force, overcome enemy defenses, isolate an element of enemy forces, and annihilate it. Then, and only then, will the Soviets advance on the next enemy element to repeat the process. We can deny this strategy if we ensure that they can never assemble sufficient forces for a COF advantage good enough for a breakthrough. Conventional offensive space capabilities give us a way to do this. Because space forces would be ''global''—in that they are available everywhere on short notice—they could deny local Soviet conventional superiority wherever they sought to gain it.

If the United States is to adopt a coherent non-nuclear strategy, it cannot ignore the Soviet conventional pillar. A number of strategic analysts are coming to the conclusion that the SDI must be expanded to include the conventional, offensive role now filled by tactical nuclear forces.[6] Fortunately, the same technology which makes it possible to counter the Soviet nuclear COF advantage can also defeat their conventional strategy.

Arms control has a key role in getting us to this non-nuclear deterrent. Unlike MAD, which would trade away the space capabilities which make this transition possible, non-nuclear arms control could usher in a new deterrent based on these capabilities. MAD would prevent us from developing these technical capabilities, and use the progress we've already reaped in the SDI as a bargaining chip to move us closer to MAD. In contrast, the strategic defender hopes to use arms control to preserve and develop these very capabilities. Once developed, the capabilities give real leverage. We could say to the Soviets, ''Look, if we deploy these systems both pillars of your grand strategy will be defunct.'' They would be faced with two evils—a costly and likely unsuccessful arms race to preserve their present strategy, or acceptance of a new deterrent relationship favorable to the West. Given traditional Soviet propensity for selecting the lesser evil, I believe they would opt for the latter. The result would be a more stable and secure world not relying on nuclear weapons. If we are skillful, we can win agreement with the Soviets without moving much beyond the development stage for the non-nuclear offensive and defensive systems I further discuss.

Disarmament: A Non-Deterrent Strategy

The fourth strategy has a growing constituency— particularly in some Western European countries. Its fundamental principle is that the Soviet threat is far less serious than the threat of war. It condemns all military approaches to national security and blames the arms, armorers, and arms bearers. Its enemy has come to be the US Government and Department of Defense. If it acknowledges a Soviet enemy, it is only those Soviet counterparts of the US military.

The strategy is one of complete disarmament. Some of its adherents propose unilateral disarmament. Their first task is to destroy all offensive arms—starting with nuclear weapons, the most threatening. In a disarmed world, they see no need for defenses and regard them as a diversion from the disarmament task at hand. The disarmers' only tool is arms control. Their dogma holds that all the West needs to do is sit down with the Soviets and convince them that we are not a threat. By example, if necessary, we should be prepared to take the first step and make concessions.

The Soviets aid and abet the disarmers. They have always advocated "complete and total disarmament." Mikhail Gorbachev, a new type of Soviet leader articulate and skilled in public relations, has been persuasive in pressing this agenda. By labeling "deterrence" the root of our adversarial problems, and claiming that arms are the source of our mutual animosity, the Soviets have won many converts in the disarmament community.

Those who espouse disarmament are sincere and their logic is straightforward. But their fundamental, and I believe irreconcilable, disagreement with the three deterrent strategies is their sanguine view of the Soviets. There may yet be an ecumenical agreement between the three deterrent schools. But I fear there can be no compromise between deterrence and complete disarmament. In the years ahead the primary debate in the United States will be between whatever deterrent school emerges and the disarmers.

Space, the Emerging Key to Military Power

In order to see how a new non-nuclear strategy makes sense, the reader should understand the impact of space capabilities on military affairs. For centuries, strategists have tried to measure and compare a new weapon's power with the old. To set the stage for later discussions, let's look briefly at how space systems stack up in these numerical measures. The results are surprising—space will soon yield greater military potential than atomic energy.

The Soviet Union itself compares space with nuclear arms in terms of potential threats to peace. While some of these statements are propaganda designed to scare Western publics into acceptance of Soviet definitions of peace, the Soviets clearly fear Western space capabilities.

Space technologies, for both offensive and defensive purposes, will soon be more potent, militarily, than nuclear weapons. I believe this is the reason for Soviet fear. Moreover, military space systems will generally lack the mass destruction "side effects" of nuclear weapons. As such, those strategies based on mass destruction, such as MAD, will be made obsolete by space technologies. This is the reason that MAD advocates, like the Soviets, avidly seek to ban the military use of space.

To show the significance of space technologies, I turn to pre-nuclear analyses. My measure of merit is "striking power." J. F. C. Fuller listed in 1945 five qualitative parameters determining a weapon's power:[7]

1. Range of action,
2. Striking power,
3. Accuracy of aim,
4. Volume of fire,
5. Portability.

Of these, he gave priority to range of action.

In the modern nuclear era, accuracy has become the key parameter.[8] Nuclear weapons release a huge amount of energy—but it is not "directed." In this case the energy density—how much energy is deposited per unit volume—falls off as the third power of distance from the explosion. Thus, a nuclear weapon which is twice as accurate is eight times as powerful as a less accurate weapon of the same explosive yield.

Fuller's first three parameters can be combined into a late 20th century parameter known as "brightness." Brightness is frequently used by laser engineers to measure the capability of a laser. But I believe it can be adapted for a more general military meaning. Brightness combines distance, accuracy, and power into a single number. It specifies how much energy the weapon puts into a cone—the physicists call this Joules (a unit of energy) per Steradian (a unit of conic volume). A Joule is about the amount of energy it takes to tap your finger on the table. A Steradian is about the size of a megaphone cone. Suppose I can hit a circle that is 10 meters in diameter and a kilometer away with an artillery shell. I first figure how many Steradians the 10-meter circle represents: $Sr = (10 \text{ Meters}/1000 \text{ meters})^2 = 10^{-4}$. If the artillery shell released 10^8 Joules when it hit, its brightness is:

$$B = 10^8 \text{ Joules}/ 10^{-4} \text{ Steradians} = 10^{12} \text{ J/Sr.}$$

Brightness alone is not a complete measure of military effectiveness. Firing rate is also important. This is why Fuller included volume of fire as a parameter. Firing rate includes two considerations: both how many "rounds" the weapon fires during a battle and how much time it takes the weapon to get into position to fire. For example, an Army unit might have 10,000 artillery rounds, but if it takes weeks to get into position (10^6 seconds), the overall firing rate would be low, averaged over the time it took to get into range and the time of the battle. In my example the final firing rate would only be 0.01/second.

The basic measure of a weapon's military power can thus be expressed:

Effectiveness = Brightness × Firing Rate.

Let me now consider weapons during the past millennia in terms of effectiveness. Table 1 lists my results and figure 2 shows them graphically. For space weapons, I address two different types, kinetic energy and directed energy weapons.[9]

The interesting result is that kinetic energy space weapons are somewhat more powerful than nuclear-armed ICBMs. But directed energy weapons in space, because they can get into position to fire rapidly, are even more powerful. I have not addressed a special kind of nuclear weapon—the so-called third generation nuclear weapon. These are weapons which use a nuclear explosion to power a directed energy weapon. However, because they are single shot devices, their effectiveness will be lower than non-nuclear directed energy weapons.[10]

The conclusion is important. Non-nuclear weapons, combined with space-basing, have more military potential than nuclear weapons. This is the reason the Soviets fear them, and this is the reason that a new deterrent relationship based on them is possible.

Table 1. Weapon Effectiveness

Era (Year AD)	Weapon	Time[a]	Brightness (J/Sr)	Firing Rate (per sec)	Effectiveness (J/Sr/sec)
1000	Arrows	6 Months	10^8	10^{-2}	10^6
1500	Bullets	3 Months	10^9	10^{-1}	10^8
1800	Artillery	1 Month	10^{12}	10^{-1}	10^{11}
1900	Artillery[b]	1 Week	10^{14}	10	10^{14}
1930	Aircraft	1 Day	10^{19}	10^{-1}	10^{18}
1950	Aircraft[c]	1 Day	10^{23}	10^{-2}	10^{21}
1970	ICBM	1 Hour	10^{23}	10^{-1}	10^{22}
2000	SBKKV[d]	1 Hour	10^{23}	10	10^{23}
2020	Laser	5 Min	10^{22}	10^2	10^{24}

[a]Time includes time of battle and time to get into position to engage.

[b]The major 19th century advance was to use rail transport to get artillery into position faster.

[c]Bomber equipped with a nuclear weapon.

[d]Space-Based Kinetic Kill Vehicle—a ''smart rock'' which destroys its target by crashing into it, i.e., with kinetic energy.

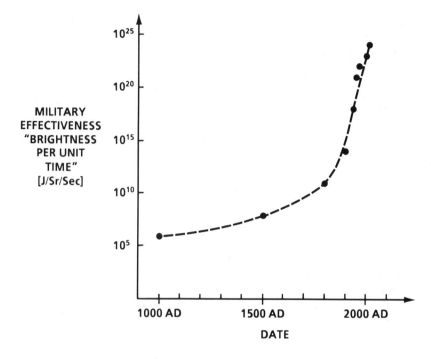

Figure 2. Increase of "Military Effectiveness" over the Past 1,000 Years. Effectiveness is defined as "brightness," or directed (aimed) destructive energy, deliverable on the enemy per unit of time.

1. VULNERABILITY-BASED NUCLEAR DETERRENCE

The average "man on the street" thinks Mutual Assured Destruction is our national nuclear strategy. While he is wrong, as I show later, we must stop and ask why the belief in MAD is so widespread. Advocates promote MAD as an immutable "fact" which we must live with. Yet, they work hard to defend MAD against alternative strategies. This argues that its logic is not as universal as its advocates proclaim. I find their arguments strongly reminiscent of a pre-nuclear discussion. I repeat this 100-year-old-plus dialogue because it typifies those I have heard in support of MAD:

> Alice tried another question. "What sort of people live about here?"
>
> "In that direction," the Cat said, waving its right paw round, "lives a hatter: and in that direction," waving the other paw, "lives a March Hare. Visit either you like: they're both mad."
>
> "But I don't want to go among mad people," Alice remarked.
>
> "Oh, you can't help that," said the Cat: "we're all mad here. I'm mad. You're mad."
>
> "How do you know I'm mad?" said Alice.
>
> "You must be," said the Cat, "or you wouldn't have come here."
>
> Conversation with the Cheshire Cat
> *Alice's Adventures in Wonderland*

MAD advocates claim the utmost in rationality, yet they argue emotionally. As an example, I list the ways in which one MAD advocate characterizes the SDI:

> "We're a hair's breadth from ultimate catastrophe."

17

"The stockpiles [are] swelled to grotesque proportions."

"The political leaders have done something supremely foolish."

"Extraordinarily dangerous, morally dubious."

"Infused with phallic imagery."

"Unbelievably perilous."

"A trillion dollars — ruinously expensive."

"Skies rippling with weapons."

"Flagrantly violates treaties."

"Tragically shortsighted and dangerous."

"Conversion of the inner solar system into a vast arena for nuclear confrontation."

Most people running across such language would assume that the commentator was a grandstanding political candidate, or, at best, a journalist for a sensationalist magazine. Not so—these remarks were made by Dr. Carl Sagan, an eminent space scientist and scholar.[1] Dr. Sagan's opinions are not isolated, but run through the writings of some of the United States' most distinguished physical scientists. What leads people from a profession known for rationality and dispassionate analysis to delve so deeply into the id for their adjectives? Why are they so sure of the path to peace in the nuclear age? How do they feel that our national security should be guaranteed?

The nation's scientists didn't waste any time after they developed the atomic bomb in 1945 in expressing their views on its meaning for international security. Leo Szilard, the physicist responsible for bringing atomic weapons to President Roosevelt's attention in 1939, wrote to the President in March 1945, three months before the atomic test at Alamogordo, New Mexico on 16 July 1945.[2] His opinion that the atomic bomb was the ultimate weapon, useful only as a means to threaten populations, was clear. In his letter to President Roosevelt he said:

Thirty million people live here in cities of over 250,000. This concentration is so pronounced that the destruction of the cities may easily mean the end of our ability to resist. Keeping constantly ahead of the Russians in our production of these heavy elements will not restore us to a strong

position. No quantity of these "active materials" which
we may accumulate will protect us from attack and so far
as retaliation is concerned, we might not be able to do
more than destroy the large cities of Russia which are few
in number and the economic importance of which is in no
way comparable to the economic importance of our own
cities. The existence of atomic bombs means the end of the
strong position of the United States in this respect. From
now on the destructive power which can be accumulated
by other countries as well as the United States can easily
reach the level at which all the cities of the "enemy" can
be destroyed in one single sudden attack.

In the moments following the Trinity test detonation, J. Robert
Oppenheimer, head of the atomic bomb project, is reported to
have said, "I have become death, the destroyer of worlds," an
excerpt from the legend of the Indian god of death, Shiva.[3] The
physicists' preoccupation with the apocalyptic nature of their
invention was pronounced from the start.

In the months following the test and subsequent use against
Hiroshima and Nagasaki, the physicists' opinions crystallized.
They made it clear that atomic bombs were useful only in
the sense that they could destroy the cities of an aggressor after
he had destroyed ours. The first issue of the *Bulletin of the
Atomic Scientists*,[4] a group formed to alert the world to the
significance of atomic weaponry, began with a somber editorial
of 7 December 1945.

Three thousand Americans—mostly members of our
Armed Forces—lost their lives in the Japanese sneak
attack. Thirty million Americans—civilians, women, and
children—may be doomed to perish if a sneak attack on
our cities by atomic bombs ever comes to pass. This catastrophe will be inevitable if we do not succeed in banishing
war from the world. Our own better preparedness could
have saved Pearl Harbor—but in a world of atomic bombs,
preparedness can only give us the power to retaliate—to
smash in our turn the cities of the nation which attacked
us.

The physicists made it equally clear that they not only thought
that defenses against atomic bombs were impossible, they were
appalled by the very idea of such defenses. When the US Navy

reported in October 1945 that a promising avenue of defense against atomic bombs was possible,[5] Dr. Szilard quickly ridiculed the idea, despite his unfamiliarity with the proposed Navy concepts.[6]

The strategic approach which the atomic physicists fathered has become known as Mutual Assured Destruction or MAD. MAD is simple. Should someone be so foolish as to start a nuclear war, a nuclear retaliation against his cities would quickly terminate his society as a functioning entity. Since the destruction would be "mutual" there would presumably be no one left to enjoy a "victory." The logic follows that it would be "mad" to trigger Mutual Assured Destruction—thus nuclear war will be tidily deterred, provided of course that everyone understands MAD and is not crazy. The MAD concept is commonly understood to have been the basis of our strategic doctrine since World War II. Even President Reagan, no enthusiast for MAD, referred to it as our current strategy.[7]

As I discuss how MAD developed, keep in mind three points about MAD:

1. Nuclear war, however destructive, is not the apocalypse, Armageddon, or absolute destruction. MAD would be better characterized as "Mutual Assured Damage."

2. Nuclear weapons are not unique in their MAD role.

3. MAD is not now, and never was, the basis of US strategy.

How MAD Developed

Although the atomic scientists invented MAD, politicians quickly adopted it. Characteristically the best description I can find of MAD is that of the greatest orator of the English language:

I must explain this term of art. "Saturation" in this connexion means the point where, although one power is stronger than the other, perhaps much stronger, both are capable of inflicting crippling or quasi-mortal injury on the other with what they have got. It does not follow, however, that the risk of war will then be greater. Indeed,

it is arguable that it will be less, for both sides will then
realize that global war would result in mutual annihilation.

                    Winston S. Churchill
                    Speech to the House of Commons
                    1955

Terror, or the threat of terror, has always been one tool in
the diplomatic and military arsenal. An interesting and, I
believe, instructive example is the Athenian discussion with and
subsequent annihilation of the Melians during the Peloponnesian
War. The Melians were allies of Sparta, Athens' mortal enemy,
who happened to live within Athens' sphere of influence. They
were offered an opportunity, under threat of annihilation, to
change allegiances, declined, and the Athenians placed them
under siege. Then, in the words of Thucydides, "The Melians
surrendered unconditionally to the Athenians, who put to death
all the men of military age they found, and sold the women and
children as slaves."[8] History is replete with similar occurrences.

The atomic bomb raised terror to center stage as an instrument of statecraft. After its development many felt that the
potential horror of nuclear war would be sufficient to usher in a
new era of world government and common good will. This attitude was particularly prevalent among the physicists who
invented the bomb, a point I will also return to several times in
this book. Serious political scientists, however, saw nuclear
weapons as a far more useful tool than merely as an inducement
for arms control. The basic precepts of terror weapons directed
against civilian populations were, interestingly enough,
developed long before the Manhattan Project by an obscure Italian aviator who wrote extensively on airpower during the 1920s.

General Giulio Douhet's now famous book, *Command of
the Air*,[9] was written in 1921, but was not widely read outside
of Italy until at least a decade later. Nevertheless, Douhet's
precepts were the basis of US and German airpower development prior to World War II. Douhet maintained that, based on
World War I experience, surface combat had reached a defensive stalemate which made war an impossibly destructive
endeavor. However, by combining airplanes with chemical (and
possibly biological) weapons, high explosive, and incendiary
bombs, warfare had undergone a "revolutionary" change. He

concluded that wars of the future would be "total," affecting and involving directly, for the first time, civilian populations.

Douhet believed that a nation could win wars by destroying the enemy population's will to resist, its manufacturing capability, and military forces on the ground. Such thinking foreshadowed the concept of a decisive preemptive attack which concerns military planners today. Douhet envisioned a strike force where ten bombers could carry sufficient bombs to destroy a circular area in an enemy city 500 meters in diameter. He concluded that a nation could destroy its enemy's cities completely in a matter of a few days. He rejected defenses against attacks, saying "there is no practical way to prevent the enemy from attacking us with his air force except to destroy his air power before he has a chance to strike at us." Douhet provided little solace to the civilian victims. "Aerial warfare admits no defense. We must therefore resign ourselves to the offensive the enemy inflicts upon us, while striving to put all our resources to work to inflict even heavier ones upon him."

Douhet also rejected past lessons, stating, "Clinging to the past will teach us nothing useful for the future, for that future will be radically different from anything that has gone before." World War II proved Douhet wrong in many ways. The bombs he said would be so destructive failed to be as effective as he had thought, civilian morale improved under bombing rather than collapsing as he had foreseen, and radar made his predictions about the efficacy of defense wrong. The most prophetic of Douhet's arguments is stated only once in his book: "The better arms are able to attack citizens in general, the more private interests are directly hurt, the fewer wars will be, for people will not be able to say anymore: Let us all arm for war, but you go and do the fighting."[10]

This fact is the basis of MAD—make war horrible enough and it won't occur. The way to make war horrible is to bring it home to the civilian population. Douhet gained some powerful adherents prior to World War II. British Prime Minister Baldwin's famous argument in 1932 that "The bomber will always get through" flowed from the idea that air power meant the potential end of civilization unless one's own air power could sufficiently threaten and deter potential enemies.[11] With the development of atomic weapons, Douhet's ideas came to the fore as the basis for national strategy, at least for Western countries.

Shortly after World War II, the United States adopted the policy that we would use our atomic might to deter aggression. It was not until 1954, though, that Secretary of State John Foster Dulles unveiled his "new look" that was to become the "Massive Retaliation" strategy of the United States. In his famous Council on Foreign Relations speech in New York on 12 January 1954, Secretary Dulles said that our method of deterring aggression, "was to depend primarily upon a great capacity to retaliate, instantly by means and at places of our choosing."[12] Saving money was our motivation for depending primarily on nuclear forces. But we also wanted to find a use for our overwhelming nuclear superiority. In actuality, the United States had relied primarily on its nuclear retaliatory might to deter war since 1945. Dulles's "new look" proved to be not so new after all.[13]

The possibility that nuclear deterrence can be mutual and a good thing was first, and probably best, stated by Bernard Brodie in the 1946 book he edited, *The Absolute Weapon*.[14] Brodie outlined the basic concept that nuclear forces on both sides would be aimed against the opponent's cities. He argued that this was a stabilizing deterrent against war which didn't have to be 100 percent credible to work as a deterrent. The risk that nuclear weapons might be introduced was sufficient for deterrence. Brodie argued that rough nuclear parity was much better than nuclear monopoly. Although he, like Douhet, rejected the concept of effective defenses against nuclear weapons, he was not so sanguine about the impossibility of war as to reject the need for some defenses. Finally, he rejected the past role of military forces as war-winning tools—preferring solely a war prevention strategy.[15]

Due to its overwhelming nuclear superiority the United States largely ignored Brodie's ideas. Not so the Western European nuclear powers. The noted British strategist, Liddell-Hart, wrote in 1947 about the impact of the atomic bomb on what he called a revolution in warfare.[16] He noted that atomic weapons, if possessed by one side only, made it essentially impossible, short of guerrilla war and other low-level combat, for anyone to start a war against that atomic power. He concluded that two sides possessing nuclear weapons made war impossible for rational states. This situation, he summed up, made international agreements to limit war both possible and imperative.

Later British analysts, most notably Sir John Slessor, Marshal of the Royal Air Force, expanded on this theme. His 1954 book, *Strategy for the West,* laid out a clear roadmap for a British MAD strategy.[17] Britain, he said, must deter Soviet adventurism through the threat of massive damage to the Soviet populace. Although Slessor regarded the Soviet Union as an evil state, he attributed rationality to Soviet leaders. If the Soviet Union could be deterred long enough, the hope of a later, more reasonable, Soviet government was worth the wait. It is not surprising that Britain, with its much smaller nuclear arsenal, came early to a policy recognizing growing Soviet power, and adopted one which did not have to match that power to have perceived utility. Churchill's famous "Balance of Terror" speech in 1955, from which the quote at the beginning of this section was taken, contains all of the elements of MAD.[18] His statement in relationship to the greatly increased destructiveness of the hydrogen bomb with regard to fission bombs (atomic bombs): "The worse things get, the better," underscores the basic MAD premise that the more horrible war can be made to seem, the more unlikely its occurrence will become. I believe that Churchill's famous closing lines best sum up the positive belief of MAD advocates:

> To conclude: mercifully, there is time and hope if we combine patience and courage. All deterrents will improve and gain authority during the next ten years. By that time, the deterrent may well reach its acme and reap its final reward. The day may dawn when fair play, love for one's fellow man, respect for justice and freedom, will enable tormented generations to march forth serene and triumphant from the hideous epoch in which we have to dwell. Meanwhile, never flinch, never weary, never despair.

France, too, as it came to possess nuclear weapons, developed a MAD strategy. Although writing as though the ideas had been developed originally in France, General Pierre

Gallois provided in his book, *The Balance of Terror*,[19] the rationale for de Gaulle's Force de Frappe. His book, published in 1962, remains the best description of the theory behind MAD. Nuclear weapons are not to be eliminated—indeed they are a most positive guarantee against war. Unlike some other strategists, he welcomed so-called tactical nuclear weapons. (Such weapons have military effectiveness similar to large conventional battlefield munitions.) By lowering the nuclear threshold and erasing the difference between nuclear and non-nuclear weapons, Gallois argued that limited wars could more easily escalate into all-out nuclear conflict. This increased risk, ironically, is positive insofar as it deters lower intensity conflict as well as general nuclear war. Gallois provided a justification for an independent nuclear force for France and Europe. He carried independence farther than most, advocating that the military commander responsible for unleashing a retaliation be independent himself from government control. This would ensure the credibility of the retaliation. He also argued that the size of a nation's retaliatory force be in proportion to the value to the Soviet Union of attacking that nation. Thus, Britain needs fewer weapons than the United States to deter an attack. Presumably, Britain also needs fewer weapons than France!

The United States was slow to consider MAD strategies. The concept of a "minimum" deterrent—which need only be large enough to devastate some proportion of Soviet cities and no more—never gained much popularity in official US policy. To be sure, the rhetoric of MAD became progressively our stated position during Secretary of Defense McNamara's tenure in the 1960s. But it never approached the "pure" form it took in Europe. Two facts led the United States to consider, but never adopt, MAD: first, the perception of Soviet nuclear parity; and second, the introduction of ballistic missiles in the early 1960s as the mainstay of Soviet nuclear power. The latter brought home the realization that the United States could suffer an attack which would be over before we could fully consider our responses.

United States strategic thought during the late 1950s and early 1960s did not focus so much on the impossibility of nuclear war, although that was generally accepted. Rather, US nuclear forces held a central, positive, and useful role in national policy. An elaborate ''game theory'' grew up around nuclear weapons, the threat to use those weapons, and the risk that military or political confrontations would result in their use. The names associated with this theory and their works are very familiar—Albert Wohlstetter, Henry Kissinger, Herman Kahn, Paul Nitze, and Thomas Schelling.[20]

The essence of MAD game theory is the game of ''chicken.'' Proposed as a sarcastic commentary on MAD by Bertrand Russell, the concept was adopted by the MAD gamesters as the basis of crisis stability analyses.[21] Chicken is an irresponsible game played by delinquent teenagers. In the game, two teenagers, each ''armed'' with an automobile, rush headlong toward one another. As mutual destruction nears, one of the players swerves—saving them both, but losing the ''chicken'' game. The winner basks in machismo victory, gaining the admiration of his peers and the affections of admiring young ladies.

Other games have also been developed to model strategic nuclear behavior. As opposed to ''chicken,'' which is a model of behavior in crises, is the game of ''prisoner's dilemma.'' An excellent description is given by Lawrence Freedman, which I summarize here.[22] Prisoner's dilemma does not deal with *crisis* stability, but rather concerns *arms race* behavior and stability. The game begins with two prisoners accused of a crime. The prosecutor orders the two separated and interrogated independently. The prisoners know that they will get the most lenient sentence if both remain silent. They have also been told that if both confess they will receive some leniency. However, if one confesses and the other does not, the stool pigeon will get off and the other prisoner will suffer the maximum penalty. Cooperation would yield the best results for both, but neither is allowed to conspire. Since each fears a double cross, a frequent result of the game is the less than optimum solution.

Countless other analogies and stability games exist (see Glen H. Snyder and Paul Diesing [23]). These games have become so arcane that I doubt that any real nuclear strategists are familiar with them.

The basis of these games is to assign numerical values, to ''quantify'' if you will, decisions nations might make on war, peace, and deterrence. From these numerical values a strategic analyst calculates whether a particular move by one side or the other makes war more likely or less likely. To illustrate the basic approach—in this case the chicken game—I set up what the analysts call a "decision matrix."

	Back Down, Soviet Union (S1)	Fight, SU (S2)
Back Down, US (U1)	U1, S1	U1, S2
Fight, US (U2)	U2, S1	U2, S2

Suppose some crisis occurs, such as the Cuban missile crisis of 1961. For this example, we imagine that there are only two options for either the Soviet Union or United States. Both nations could fight for their position, the Soviet Union to keep its missiles in Cuba, the United States to have them removed. Similarly, either side could back down. Each side would assign some numerical value to the two options. For the United States the willingness to fight could get the missiles out and lower the long-term threat to US security as well as strengthen its reputation for toughness. These considerations might have been very important to us in 1961 and on a scale of 100 we would assign a willingness to fight a 60. Thus, $U2 = 60$. We could also have seen some value in backing down since that would lower the immediate chance of a confrontation which might lead to global nuclear war. For the United States that was probably a lesser concern in 1961, so $U1 = 40$. The Soviet Union might have seen the situation differently. Although the prestige of getting their way in Cuba would have been a plus, the risk of nuclear war with what was then a much stronger United States might have been far more important. The Soviet Union could have assigned a value of willingness to fight, $S2 = 20$, and a value of backing down and avoiding nuclear war risk, $S1 = 80$. The decision matrix, filled out, thus looks as follows:

	Back Down, SU	Fight, SU
Back Down, US	40, 80	40, 20
Fight, US	60, 80	60, 20

When the analysts add up the numbers, the possibility which had the the greatest combined value, in this case the United States getting its way and the Soviet Union backing down, is most probable.

MAD is particularly appealing because it represents an absolute bound to the problem—namely "the end of the world." Games have far more meaning when there are such absolute boundaries. For this reason, analysts tend to prefer MAD.

Thomas Schelling's 1966 book *Arms and Influence*[24] marked a high point in MAD game theory. Its basic approach was to consider how the potential to inflict pain, as opposed to the actual act itself, is a tool of international diplomacy short of war. Thus, although actual nuclear weapons use is forbidden, these weapons, by existing, are still useful. Schelling noted numerous examples of state-sponsored terrorism as an instrument of policy, including various "pacification" campaigns against the American Indians. However, he perceived some essential differences between those non-nuclear terrorist actions and nuclear weapons. In particular:

1. Nuclear weapons can inflict mass death quickly, distinguishing them from older weapons.

2. Because of the ease in delivering nuclear weapons, one side can inflict mass death on the other even if its army is losing on the battlefield. Prior to nuclear weapons it was possible to kill most of an enemy's population, but you had to first defeat his army in battle. Nuclear weapons eliminate this requirement.

Schelling's ideas added a number of interesting twists to previous work. To use potential pain as a weapon, you must become concerned with your enemy's intentions more than with his military forces. Thus, detailed military balance of forces matters little. The element of risk, as in Russell's chicken game, is all-important. Protagonists can manipulate risk and uncertainty. Ironically, the type of unpredictability exhibited by Hitler prior to World War II can be a positive asset. Another "asset" is to place oneself in the position where retreat is politically difficult if not impossible—that is, burn the bridges behind one's army. Schelling made a significant distinction between "deterrence" and "compellence." Deterrence is persuading a potential enemy not to do something, while compellence is persuading him to do something. United States "deterrent" policy has contained elements of both.

Schelling's (and similar) work in the late 1950s and early 1960s marked a change in US thinking. Public officials increasingly used the rhetoric of MAD, while the strategic theorists were concluding that we needed a far more sophisticated strategy than simply threatening to blow up the world. Facts show that we never adopted MAD instead of the sophisticated "retaliation-based" warfighting deterrent I will discuss in the next chapter.

To be sure, theorists like Schelling made many simplifications. First, the theories assumed international relations take place between two rational actors, or, as some critics called it, the "rationality of the irrational."[25] To place this in the context of Graham Allison's models for decisionmaking, the "rational actor" model treats states as single rational individuals.[26] Allison also identified models based on equally valid bureaucratic-tradition forces and the personalities of the individual leaders within the hierarchy. Second, as Schelling admitted, strategic models ignore issues of morality. While acknowledging the basic immorality of bargaining with mass murder threats, Schelling noted that moral squeamishness is counterproductive to the bargaining process. In short, like most strategists, Schelling forgot that we are the "good" guys. Third, nuclear weapons themselves present a logical dilemma. In order for MAD to work, adversaries must believe that the other side might actually use nuclear weapons in some situations. But the basis of MAD is that nuclear weapons are fundamentally different—so different that their use would mean the end of the world. MAD requires not only the existence of unusable weapons but the belief that someone might actually use them. A strange game indeed!

History has much to say about MAD and post-MAD reasoning, despite the erroneous view that there is no relevant history prior to 16 July 1945. Schelling's view that assured destruction could not be accomplished until the destruction of the enemy's armed forces prior to 1945 is contradicted by history. It has never been necessary to have totally defeated the enemy, in order to visit mass destruction on its population. There are numerous examples where civilian populations were annihilated even while their military forces were winning victories far from home.

How much assured destruction is enough? To get right to the dirty work, it must be understood that even a global, full nuclear war would *not*, I repeat would *not* be the end of mankind, would *not* be the end of civilization, would *not* be the end of the principal combatants, and even would *not* be an event of "unparalleled" destruction. Others who have made these points have been vilified. Nonetheless, the statements are true.

In his 1960 work, *On Thermonuclear War*,[27] Herman Kahn considered the effects of nuclear war on the United States. He concluded that while nuclear war would be a disaster for the United States, it would not be an "unlimited" one. He made this point by considering the nation to be two separate countries, which he called country "A," and country "B." Country "A" holds the urban and industrial centers, country "B" holds the rural and dispersed industrial elements. Kahn acknowledged that a nuclear war might destroy most, if not all, of country "A." However, virtually any conceivable nuclear war would leave country "B" largely intact. Country "B" could then provide the nucleus for national recovery. Kahn also pointed out that deaths, even in country "A," could be limited and economic recovery accelerated by modest civil defense measures, particularly some protection against radioactive fallout. For suggesting that nuclear war might not be Armageddon, Kahn was chastised by the scientific community. The *Scientific American* review of his book called it "a moral tract on mass murder: how to plan it, how to conduct it, how to get away with it, how to justify it." That 1961 review was less delicate in its conclusion, "this evil and tenebrous book, with its loose-lipped pieties and its hayfoot-strawfoot logic, is permeated with a bloodthirsty irrationality such as I have not seen in my years of reading."[28]

Kahn was not alone in forfeiting the approval of the scientific community. In 1982, Deputy Under Secretary of Defense for Strategic and Theater Nuclear Forces, Thomas ("T.K.") Jones, told a newspaper reporter that, "If there are enough shovels to go around, everybody's going to make it."[29] His simple civil defense means, primarily covering a small part or corner of one's house with a few feet of dirt, are very similar to Soviet civil defense efforts and could be highly effective. Jones' comments were met with ridicule in the scientific community.

Partially as a result of renewed interest in nuclear war survival, some members of the scientific community prepared a doomsday concept—nuclear winter. These calculations "proved" that nuclear war would trigger an ice age which would end all life on earth. The nuclear winter concept became a major issue in the mid-1980s. Careful scientific analysis of nuclear winter's assumptions showed them to be seriously flawed.[30] The fact that the nuclear winter theory was never scientifically reviewed prior to publication, and was quickly used in political attacks on Administration strategic policy, has led some to charge that it was deliberately fabricated by scientists hoping to force the politicians into accepting MAD.[31] The length to which scientific vigor is "prostituted" in service of political goals has become increasingly disturbing—as I show later in this chapter for the case of so-called scientific criticisms of SDI. The public has heard far more favorable scientific comment on the technically unsupportable nuclear winter theory than on the well-founded civil defense arguments of T. K. Jones.

How Much Destruction?

How many people would die in a global nuclear war? This question is, of course, controversial and uncertain. However, I have been able to find general agreement in several calculations. The best calculations avoid strategic and moral musings. A good example is Carl F. Miller's 1970 study, *Assessment of Nuclear Weapons Requirements for Assured Destruction.*[32] That study agreed with Kahn's 1960 conclusion that the United States can be divided into urban and non-urban elements for the purposes of nuclear war damage analysis. Miller reported that about 60 percent of the population and 80 percent of US manufacturing is concentrated in several thousand places with populations greater than 2500 people. All studies I reviewed agreed that this "urban" component is targetable and the rest of the US population is essentially not. Miller's study, a 1964 DOD study on which McNamara based his MAD requirements,[33] and a 1985 Congressional Office of Technology Assessment report[34] all showed that urban population density, except for a few of the most densely populated central city areas, is about 3000 people per square mile. I can therefore derive a very simple mathematical relation for the number of people killed in an attack:

$$\text{percent population destroyed} = \frac{\text{square miles destroyed} \times 3000}{\text{US population (240 million in 1985)}}$$

The 1964 DOD report showed that roughly the same relation holds for the Soviet Union. However, only one-third of the Soviet population is urban in contrast to the two-thirds US urban fraction. Conversely, Soviet industry is more concentrated than US industry. Eighty percent of Soviet industry is in urban areas—the same fraction which is co-located with the larger US urban population.

The rural population of both countries is essentially untargetable. For example, Miller calculated that some four million nuclear warheads would be needed to approach complete destruction of the US population. Thus, "total" destruction of the United States or Soviet Union is not possible.

In addition to the "prompt" effects of a nuclear war, primarily the nuclear blast and associated fires, there are also "delayed" nuclear effects. The principal delayed effects are radioactive fallout and possible long-term environmental problems—nuclear winter.

The basic measure of blast effects is "overpressure" measured in pounds per square inch. To place this measure in context, the earth's atmosphere exerts about 15-pounds-per-square-inch pressure, which means there are about 1000 pounds pushing against your face every second of every day. The reason your face doesn't collapse is that an equal pressure pushing from the blood, air and flesh pushes from inside your face. An explosion, nuclear or otherwise, adds pressure on the outside that cannot readily be balanced from the inside—so damage occurs. A few pounds overpressure is like getting a good stiff punch in the nose. The farther away from an explosion the lower the overpressure—overpressure falls off dramatically with distance, specifically with the cubed power of distance. A few pounds overpressure will damage buildings—blowing out windows and the like. A wooden building will collapse at about 10 pounds overpressure, but reinforced concrete buildings can take 20-50 pounds overpressure and remain standing. Nuclear weapons also produce intense heat. The heat associated with about five pounds overpressure is sufficient to set wooden buildings afire.

The levels of overpressure needed to kill are vigorously argued, with the only empirical data coming from Hiroshima and Nagasaki. Miller cited studies of these blasts which showed some deaths at about two pounds overpressure, 50 percent dead at 15 pounds overpressure, and everyone dead when there's more than 20 pounds overpressure.

The maximum blast damage against a city occurs in an "air burst," where the nuclear weapon detonates a few thousand feet above ground. The area "destroyed" depends on what one considers that word to mean. I believe that a fair meaning of destruction is the area in which over half the people are killed by the blast. Based on the Hiroshima and Nagasaki data, those deaths occurred at 15 pounds overpressure. I can thus derive a simple equation for area destroyed as a function of weapon yield:

Destroyed area (square miles) $= \pi \times 0.0507 \times$ (kilotons of TNT)$^{2/3}$. I can combine these results with the earlier relationship to figure out how many people would be killed in an attack specifically aimed at cities:

$$\frac{\text{Percent}}{\text{killed}} = \frac{\text{Number of bombs} \times \pi \times 0.0507 \times (\text{yield in KT})^{2/3} \times 3000}{\text{US Population (240 million in 1985)}}$$

In addition to the blast and fire effects, delayed radiation-induced deaths can be high in number. Miller's study reports that radiation from a surface burst, which gives less blast damage but much more radiation, can contaminate a lethal area ten times larger than the lethal blast area from a similar-sized air burst. However, protection against radiation is possible. Staying inside your house can double your chances of surviving radiation effects. A moderate concrete shelter can decrease radiation effects a hundred-fold. Fallout-related deaths with such protection would be confined to an area smaller than blast-related deaths. From such calculations, T.K. Jones derived his reasonable recommendation that people surviving a nuclear blast could protect themselves from fallout through simple means, such as staying in the basement for the few weeks necessary for the fallout to subside to tolerable levels.

If the "end of humanity" is not in the cards, what constitutes sufficient destruction to ensure mutual deterrence? This value is very much in the eye of the beholder. Curiously, MAD strategists have lowered the ante with time. Defense Secretary McNamara's 1965, 1967, and 1969 budget statements to Congress made a stab at what constitutes MAD.[35] These numbers progressively decreased. In 1965, the death of one-third of the Soviet population was considered an appropriate deterrent. By 1969, this figure had dropped to one-fifth. A 1985 article, co-authored by Secretary McNamara and Hans Bethe, a physicist who worked on the Manhattan Project, states that 1,000 warheads would be sufficient.[36] My equation translates that into about one-tenth of the Soviet population—the same percentage given in the 1985 Office of Technology Assessment report. McNamara was a technical adviser for that report and I assume that he endorsed that conclusion. I might add, a bit facetiously, that this trend would result in zero percent casualties assuring destruction by the early 1990s.

Is this assured destruction an "unbounded" or even "unprecedented" calamity warranting somber references to Armageddon or the apocalypse? If all warheads in both Soviet and US arsenals were targeted against cities and industrial areas, roughly half the US population, and a third of the Soviet population would perish. Because US arsenals and, we believe, Soviet arsenals are not targeted primarily against population centers, casualties might be a factor of two lower than these worst-case estimates.

Is McNamara's 10 percent population loss, or, for that matter, today's worst-case possibility an unimaginable catastrophe? History suggests it is not. Herman Kahn pointed out that the Soviet Union lost ten percent of its population and thirty percent of its industry in World War II—not to mention the previous 15 years of "socialization" during which Stalin inflicted a similar number of casualties in furthering development of "the worker's paradise."[37] Thus, while nuclear war qualifies for the Soviet Union as horrible and probably even a catastrophe, it is not unprecedented.

Can a nation recover from nuclear war? Popular literature and movies such as On the Beach[38] (1957) and The Day After[39] (1984) say not. Nuclear war would not return us to the Stone Age as Winston Churchill suggested—nor even "hurl [us] ten centuries

into the past'' as General Pierre Gallois claimed.[40] Figure 3
shows economic development for the last fifty years of
the major industrial nations.[41] Even those nations hardest hit
by World War II recovered in about a decade. Herman Kahn
showed data indicating that for each 10 percent of the population lost in a war, about a decade additional is needed for
recovery.[42] There are, to use Kahn's words, "tragic but dis-
tinguishable postwar states."

   Skeptics may point out that these numbers have no meaning because we can never truly know the full interlocking
impact of losing half a population. Without tarrying too long on
the macabre, we do have a historical example of mass death on
the scale of nuclear war—the Black Death of the late Middle
Ages. Between 1347 and 1350, about 25 to 45 percent of Europe

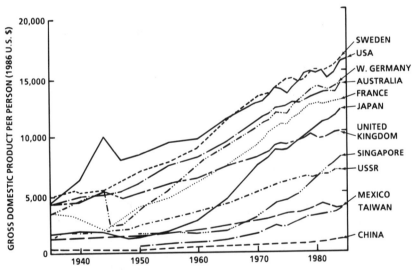

Source: Derived from *Report of the National Commission on Space* (New York:
Bantam, 1986), p. 185.

**Figure 3. Growth in Gross Domestic Product for Major Indus-
trialized States.** Note the rapid recovery of Germany and Japan following World War II. These nations lost a sizable fraction of their
industry during the war. Although Soviet losses during this period
were as bad or worse than Germany and Japan, overall Soviet domestic product appears to have been little affected by the war.

perished; Pope Clement IV calculated in 1351 that 23,840,000 died out of Europe's population of about 75 million. Experts on the subject suggest that European population would have returned to pre-plague levels in three decades—consistent with Herman Kahn's nuclear war calculations. However, the plague returned to Europe about once a decade for more than a century—equivalent to having a major nuclear war every ten years. Between 1349 and 1450 Europe's population fell by 60-75 percent.[43]

The scientific community has not welcomed these facts. The US Civil Defense structure has pointed out the thoughts I outlined above. For example in 1979 the government stated: "Even under the worst circumstances imaginable there is no danger of a repetition of the Bubonic Plague that devastated Europe in the mid-14th century, or other types of potentially catastrophic epidemics."[44]

The physical science community ridicules these statements, but offers no technical rebuttal. For example, a *Bulletin of the Atomic Scientists* critique of programs for surviving nuclear war dismisses these points with: "The Black Death, which claimed the lives of perhaps one-third the population of Europe over a three-year period, left the cities standing, the rural infrastructure in place, the environment unscathed. World War II killed perhaps 30-40 million people over a six-year period, but the assaults occurred in stages; some areas could recover to help those more recently affected; and there always remained an outside."[45]

In fact, these arguments are unconvincing. There was essentially no industrial base in medieval Europe. Nuclear war today would leave the rural infrastructure in place, as I have said earlier, and would also leave much of the world, even perhaps much of the industrial world, largely intact.

I have not presented this discussion to earn a reputation for bloody-mindedness, although I will surely be accused of that. Rather, we should understand the degree to which hyperbole over strategic matters has taken over. The exaggeration of nuclear consequences is widespread. If our potential adversaries do not share the same capacity for self-terror, we could be in serious trouble. The epidemic of exaggeration has spread from the scientific community to the military. Comments from the military establishment in the late 1940s cautioned reason with regards to nuclear weapons and nuclear war, unlike the scientists. Occasionally, however, we hear a statement like that made in 1981 by General David Jones, Chairman of the Joint Chiefs of Staff: "If all weapons were targeted in such a way as to give maximum damage to urban and industrial areas, you are talking about the greatest catastrophe in history by many orders of magnitude."[46] General Jones had surely seen briefings similar to the one I saw on nuclear war outcomes and he must have known that such a summary judgment was highly debatable. Nonetheless, the public tends to believe an official of his stature. Further, such questionable views are reinforced daily by the scientific community and popular press.

Does MAD Require Nuclear Weapons?

Many who passionately desire the end of nuclear weapons fear what may replace them. Perhaps they recall stories read as children, such as H.G. Wells's *The War of the Worlds*:

> It is still a matter of wonder how the Martians are able to slay men so swiftly and so silently.... However it is done, it is certain that a beam of heat is the essence of the matter. Heat, and invisible, instead of visible, light. Whatever is combustible flashes into flame at its touch, lead runs like water, it softens iron, cracks and melts glass, and when it falls upon water, incontinently that explodes into steam.

Some critics of the current move toward strategic defenses fear giant "Death Star" spaceships hovering over the planet, ready to zap everyone with death rays. The attitude of many is to live with the nuclear devil for fear of something much worse. The Outer Space Treaty, signed in 1967, outlaws the placing in space of "nuclear weapons or other kinds of weapons of mass destruction."[47] The Treaty and its negotiating record did not elaborate on what these "other" weapons were.

In writings since 1945, the possibility of non-nuclear weapons as destructive as their nuclear counterparts was occasionally raised. Biological weapons are sometimes lumped with nuclear weapons, particularly in earlier writings. For example, Max Lerner's 1962 book, *The Age of Overkill*, notes some similar effects of biological and nuclear weapons.[48] However, most writings ignore the mass-destruction potential of chemical and biological weapons. A notable exception to this trend occurs in writings from more conservative strategists who reject the principles of MAD. For example, the conservative Institute for Foreign Policy Analysis (IFPA) in Cambridge, MA published a pamphlet in 1984 pointedly entitled, *CBW: The Poor Man's Atomic Bomb*.[49] MAD strategists appear strangely reluctant to apply "nuclear" logic to non-nuclear possibilities. This tendency probably results from desires to preserve the MAD precept that nuclear weapons are fundamentally different.

General Douhet, whom I showed earlier to be the "grandfather," if not the father of MAD, based his 1921 analysis on the combined destructive effects of explosives, incendiaries, and chemical weapons. He also noted the potential role of biological weapons. Douhet envisioned explosives breaking apart buildings, incendiaries lighting them afire, and chemical weapons preventing firefighters from combating the flames. The Italian general calculated that 10 tons of explosives could destroy a circle within a city 500 meters in diameter (one third of a square mile). This, he claimed was "scientifically" proven. Indeed, the 1942 translation of Douhet notes that the 15 November 1940 German raid on Coventry proved Douhet correct. Douhet said that the 10-ton munition load could be delivered by a 10-bomber strike force and envisioned a national strike force of 1000 bombers. This force, according to Douhet, could destroy 50 cities a day, and 1000 tons of bombs delivered in a single day could wipe out the largest cities of the time, London and Paris. The key to this ability to wipe out an enemy's society was the "revolutionary" nature of poison gas and aircraft.

Douhet identified all of the elements of MAD. Referring back to my nuclear destruction equations, each of Douhet's 10-bomber strike forces had the destructive potential of a several kiloton weapon—a typical tactical nuclear weapon in today's arsenals. Ten such units are equivalent to one of today's 100-kiloton strategic warheads. Moreover, the poison gas element of

Douhet's bombs provides the same "delayed" effects as radio-active fallout. Douhet's view that enemy societies would be destroyed in a day or so is another key element of MAD.

Current commentators give General Douhet the credit for inventing MAD, but note that his predictions needed the destructiveness of nuclear weapons to bring them to reality (see, for example Schell's book, *The Abolition*[50]). Actual bombing experience in World War II, despite Coventry, tended to invalidate Douhet's predictions. Herman Kahn pointed out that German calculations prior to World War II overrated conventional bombing destructiveness by a factor of ten.[51]

The fact remains that chemical weapons could perform an "assured destruction" mission against unprotected civilian populations. During World War II, Germany developed the "nerve" gases Sarin and Soman. Sarin (GB) is the principal nerve agent in US arsenals. Nerve gas has the effect on people that commercial bug sprays have on insects. In addition to those nerve gases which must be inhaled to kill, the United States has developed VX—a nerve agent absorbed through the skin which is lethal even in small quantities. According to reports presented during an international conference sponsored by the Carnegie Foundation in 1977, VX is "lethally dangerous from a matter of days to weeks"[52]—similar to the lethal period for radioactive fallout from nuclear weapons. The Carnegie report stated that a single ground attack aircraft could lethally contaminate a square mile, and that four tons of nerve agent could kill several thousand people if used in urban areas.[53]

From these data, I adopt the rough relationship that one ton of nerve agent can lethally contaminate a square mile—about equivalent to the Hiroshima atomic bomb. If the current Soviet SS-18 ICBM were loaded with VX, at eight tons per missile, then the Soviet SS-18 force of about 300 missiles could "destroy" 2400 square miles of US urban territory. From the curves provided in the aforementioned Office of Technology Assessment report, this strike would kill, if optimally targeted, about 10 percent of the US population (20 million). This is the number which Secretary McNamara and the Congressional Office of Technology Assessment seem to believe is sufficient for MAD.

Biological agents and toxins (chemical poisons produced by microorganisms—but which must be ingested to kill), are even more potent than nerve agents. Bacteria (such as anthrax) are 100 times more potent per pound than nerve agents.[54] In 1960 Major General Marshall Stubbs, head of the US Army Chemical Corps, said that 10 aircraft armed with biological agents could kill or *incapacitate* 30 percent of the US population.[55] To accomplish as much with nuclear weapons requires about 10,000 nuclear warheads—three times the current Soviet SS-18 force. With a lethality ratio of 20 pounds of anthrax per square mile, *three SS-18s could guarantee MAD against our country*. Lest the reader dismiss these calculations as unfounded, biological weapons have, like nuclear weapons and Douhet's bombs, some empirical data. The IFPA report revealed that a "test" was conducted against San Francisco in the 1950s. A "benign" bacteria was released over the city from boats offshore. Subsequent analysis showed that essentially everyone in the city had inhaled at least 5000 bacteria. Had these bacteria been pneumonic plague, a form of Black Death, more than 80 percent of the city's population would have died.

Based on the efficiency of these "bugs and drugs," one must wonder why the superpowers have not dumped their nuclear arsenals in favor of a far more cost-effective bacteriological deterrent. The reason cannot be lack of knowledge among military planners, since an old medieval siege trick was to catapult a few dead horses over the city wall to induce epidemics among the besieged populace. The arms control lobby in the United States must fear this logic because they approach the topic in only the most oblique way. The Carnegie conference only touched on this subject once, saying: "Computer simulations suggest that, in terms of expected casualties per ton of munitions, they [nerve agents] would be somewhat more powerful than massed incendiaries when used in large-scale attacks against urban populations."[56]

The reason nations don't depend on chemical and biological weapons (CBW) deterrents to enforce MAD is, as I emphasize throughout this book, that MAD doesn't work. Those weapons, despite their lethality against civilian populations, are not very cost-effective military weapons, particularly against hardened military targets. Quite simply, they are militarily impotent and obsolete.

If CBWs are not good for MAD, are there others? Soviet propagandists have attempted to suggest that directed energy weapons (lasers) would make good mass destruction weapons. The Soviet position at the November 1985 summit focused on the mass destruction potential of lasers—probably in the hopes of invoking the 1967 Outer Space Treaty provisions against such weapons. Some US "experts" have, perhaps unwittingly, supported Soviet ideas. Characteristically, a Soviet document handed out during the 1985 summit gave full and sole credit for these ideas to the West: "It has been reported in the American press that space-strike weapons could also hit ground and sea targets."[57]

In May 1985, two physicists, Albert Latter and Ernest Martinelli, published a paper suggesting that missile defense laser weapons placed in space would themselves have assured destruction potential.[58] Most ballistic missile defense weapons (particle beams, homing rockets, and nuclear-powered lasers) cannot penetrate the atmosphere and therefore have no potential against ground targets. However, some types of lasers can reach the surface of earth from space. Latter and Martinelli's paper examined a situation with 500 laser platforms in orbit as the heart of a global ballistic missile defense system. They postulated that these lasers, optimally configured, could in the course of several hours light tens of millions of fires in urban areas, triggering fire storms as devastating as a nuclear attack, although there are a variety of technical uncertainties which could invalidate their conclusions. This paper was the basis of Soviet propaganda and domestic criticism of strategic defense-reliant deterrent relationships.[59]

According to Dr. Gregory Canavan of the Los Alamos National Laboratory, it is theoretically possible to ignite a fire storm with space-based lasers.[60] The type of laser envisioned by Latter and Martinelli could start a fire on a building's roof, or even through windows on combustible material. The area ignited would be about a foot across. The amount of energy needed to start a fire is about 10-45 kilojoules—similar to the energy in a 4th of July firecracker or a book of matches. The latter similarity is not insignificant, because a few thousand KGB agents armed with matchbooks could probably start as many fires and with as great an effect as the space lasers. A space laser system might be able to start up to 100 million fires under extremely optimistic circumstances.

Could a Soviet space laser system light the United States afire? Canavan says yes—with some important caveats. Curiously enough, it is almost exclusively US *suburban* areas which have a high enough density of combustible targets to produce a fire storm. US urban areas and almost all Soviet population centers are non-combustible concrete and masonry. Yet, the possibility of igniting US neighborhoods, using lasers, is less important than the cost-effectiveness of such actions and countermeasures against such an attempt.

Table 2 lists some assumptions on laser costs and costs for a nuclear offensive system. The key point to take from this chart is that the cost per pound of TNT equivalent delivered on target is $25 million for the laser system. Nuclear weapons deliver the same 1-pound TNT equivalent for about two cents. Unlike biological weapons, lasers fail in mass-destruction cost effectiveness by about a factor of one billion. Ironically, more energy could be delivered against the United States by crashing the laser platforms into the ground than from the laser beam energy.

It is important to calculate the detailed cost effectiveness, not only of delivering energy, but also of igniting a fire storm. A 100-kiloton warhead can, in principle, start fires down to overpressures of 5 pounds per square inch covering an area of

Table 2. Strategic System Data

Strategic Offensive Systems

Warhead Yield:	500 Kilotons TNT
Warhead Costs:	$20 Million apiece

Laser Defensive Systems (estimates)

Power Output:	25 Megawatts*
Laser Operation Time:	150 Seconds
Laser Orbital Altitude:	1000 Kilometers
Deliverable Laser Energy:	1 Ton TNT
Laser Platform Cost:	$500 Million apiece

*Laser power is measured in joules per second or "watts." A joule is a unit of energy and a watt is a unit of power. A 25-megawatt laser puts out the equivalent of about 10 kilograms of TNT every second.

30 square miles—an area about ten times greater than the total destruction zone from blast effects alone. If the Soviets wanted to ignite fires to affect one-third of the US population, they would need about 1000 nuclear warheads to cover the 30,000-odd square miles occupied by 80 million people—for a total cost of about $20 billion. The same job done with the laser system is at least ten times more expensive. Of course, if the laser system were exhausted attacking enemy cities, it would not be available for its primary job—defending the nation from nuclear weapons.

In addition to cost-effectiveness problems, there are simple countermeasures to laser-induced firestorms. For example, a thin layer of non-combustible paint sprayed over combustible surfaces would largely eliminate a building's vulnerability. Tests done during the 1950s showed that even a thin layer of *combustible* paint doubled resistance to nuclear-induced fires. The cost of fire retardant is a tiny fraction of a laser system. An even simpler countermeasure would be to tell the spouse to be on the lookout for laser attacks and to keep a bucket of water by the door. If the occupants of a house hear a laser strike they would quickly climb to the roof and douse the small smouldering spot before it spreads to the rest of the house. I conclude that mass destruction using lasers need not worry us for the foreseeable future.

Are there other mass destruction weapons on the horizon? Some space-weapon critics have suggested that the military be kept out of space for fear they will throw rocks.[61] A famous science fiction story of the 1950s, Robert Heinlein's *The Moon is a Harsh Mistress*, had military forces based on the moon threatening the planet with mass destruction from moon rocks crashing to earth.[62] These seemingly ridiculous ideas have some basis in reality.* The famous meteor crater in Arizona is dramatic proof that big rocks from space (about 1 million tons) can equal the largest nuclear weapons (100 megatons) in destructiveness. To compare the destructiveness of nuclear weapons ($E = mc^2$) with these kinetic energy ($E = 1/2mv^2$) weapons is simple. Four thousand tons of rock (about 30 feet on a side) traveling at ten miles

---

* For, as I showed in the introduction, space capabilities will soon match, and then exceed, nuclear weapons in *military* potential.

per second—the velocity it would have if "dropped" from the moon, has the same energy as a 100-kiloton bomb. But, cost-effectiveness arguments again show the infeasibility of this approach. During the 1983 Defensive Technologies Study, which formed the basis of the President's Strategic Defense Initiative, I commissioned a study on how cheaply lunar and other near-earth resources could be returned to earth.[63] Dollar costs about 10 percent of current launch cost appeared possible in the next 50 years—maybe $100 per pound. With these costs, a moon-rock bomb, hardly a covert first-strike weapon, would cost roughly $1 billion, compared with current nuclear warhead costs of about $20 million. Again, exotic *mass destruction* weapons are theoretically feasible, but economically and militarily impractical. While space weapons have great military potential, they have little mass-destruction capability for the foreseeable future. These proposals, put forth in a serious vein, remind me of the oft-told story of the scientist during World War II who developed an effective counter to the German U-boat menace. He proposed boiling the oceans!

I am led to the following three propositions:

1. Assured destruction existed long before nuclear weapons. Moreover, nuclear weapons are not the only way to produce assured destruction.

2. Cost-effectiveness analyses suggest that nuclear weapons have not been chosen as the mainstay of our arsenals based on their assured destruction potential. Other weapons could do that more cheaply.

3. Exotic space-related technologies will not, despite assertions by critics, usher us into a new era of ever more destructive weapons.

The Role of Defenses in MAD

If anyone can prove to me that we could *surely* and *completely* protect our country from eventual aero-chemical offensives by means of a determined organized aerial defense, practically possible to bring into existence, I am ready to give up all my theories.

General Giulio Douhet
Command of the Air, 1921

MAD's basic premise is a world faced with *infinitely* destructive offensive weapons. From this assumption it follows in elementary mathematical simplicity that there can be no defense. I can quantify the gain my military actions achieve against an enemy and the loss his actions inflict upon me as follows.

$$W \text{ (net gain or loss)} = (O_{us} - D_{enemy}) - (O_{enemy} - D_{us})$$

where O and D represent offensive and defense effectiveness respectively for us and the enemy. If W comes out positive for us, that is victory, and if it comes out negative, that is defeat. It is clear that an "infinite" offense, whether nuclear or otherwise, on both sides means that both sides lose regardless. The conclusion, in the words of a warfighting computer in the recent movie *War Games* is, "The only way to win is not to play." Adherents of MAD believe this relationship is so simple that those ignoring it must be either crazy or stupid. It must be concluded, these advocates assert, that anyone desiring defenses in the face of this logic must either (1) not believe that offensive damage is infinite, i.e., must be crazy, or (2) can't see that finite defense against infinite offense is a waste of money, i.e., must be stupid.

Douhet made his disdain of defensive weapons clear—"we cannot dig trenches in the air." He rejected defensive efforts with two special exceptions. The first was the defensive use of offensive forces: "There is no practical way to prevent an enemy from attacking us with his air force except to destroy his airpower before he has a chance to strike us." Despite this caveat, Douhet believed that attacks against the enemy's armed forces were secondary: "The objective in war has never at any time been the enemy's armed forces. It has always been, is now, and always will be to win. In the future, war will be waged against the unarmed population of the cities and great industrial centers."[64]

Douhet also allowed another "defensive" mission, the "point" defense of exceptionally valuable targets such as air bases. All of the assumptions of MAD were thus in place in the 1920s:

1. Countervalue attacks against enemy populations are the principal objective.

2. Counterforce attacks against military forces are useful as damage limiting means, but secondary to countervalue operations.

3. Point defense can be useful to deny an enemy counterforce results.

4. Area defenses of the population are technically impossible.

So firmly ingrained were these offense-dominant ideas prior to World War II that hauntingly familiar arguments abounded. There were the famous Stanley Baldwin-Winston Churchill debates in Britain with Churchill urging air defense efforts and Baldwin firmly asserting that "The bomber will always get through."[65] Misleading calculations of the infeasibility of defense were commonplace. For example, a 1941 discussion by Fletcher Pratt in the United States just prior to our entry into the war concluded that 120,000 antiaircraft guns manned by 4,200,000 men would be needed to defend just the northeastern US cities from air attack—an attempt Pratt concluded was "absurd."[66]

World War II convinced US military planners that defensive efforts, both point and area, were feasible and essential— even against atomic weapons. The V-1 and V-2 attacks against London failed for defensive reasons. Herman Kahn pointed out that the British succeeded in shooting down 24 percent of the V-1s in the first week of the attack. Just before German cessation of these attacks, the British were able to shoot down 95 percent of the V-1s. The V-2s to which the Germans turned and against which there was no defense were not cost-effective in the damage they did versus their economic cost to Germany.[67]

In a remarkably prescient discussion of the future, General of the Air Force, H.H. ("Hap") Arnold, foresaw ICBMs and even space-based nuclear weapons at the end of the war. Despite these new developments, against which no defense seemed forthcoming, General Arnold advocated intense efforts to find such defenses. He also placed bomber defense on an equal priority to our offensive efforts.[68]

Advice from military quarters on the value of such defenses was ignored and even ridiculed by the budding nuclear strategists of the late 1940s. Bernard Brodie's hallmark 1946 essays in *The Ultimate Weapon* repeatedly stressed that defense against nuclear weapon attack was both unlikely and undesirable.[69] Brodie particularly took military and political leaders to task for suggesting that they were feasible and should be pursued. Among those chastised were President Truman, Admiral Nimitz, and General McNaughton (Canadian Chief of Staff). Brodie believed the only way defense could play an effective role was for it to be perfect—a technical impossibility. Brodie also began a hallowed tradition of citing scientists in support of his contentions. To his credit, he also expressed skepticism on the scientists' dispassion toward the subject of nuclear war.

The inventors of the atomic bomb wasted no time, as I noted at the beginning of this chapter, in insisting that atomic defense was impossible. When the Navy reported that it might have found an atomic bomb defense in October 1945, Dr. Leo Szilard, one of the physicists who had written President Roosevelt in 1945 on the possibility of atomic weapons while admitting that he did not know any details, said six days later "If someone invented a device to do that I would undertake to develop within fifteen minutes a counter defense; that is, a defense against that defense."[70]

As Robert McNamara progressively declared a MAD policy in the 1960s, he increasingly rejected the possibility of defense. In his 1963 Statement to Congress, he placed top priority on strategic defense, saying, "The most urgent problem confronting us in the Continental Air and Missile Defense Forces is defense against ICBM attack."[71] But, in his last statement to Congress he had completely changed his tune, rejecting all but perfect defense for populations and cities, stating, "This is not simply a matter of technology, it is inherent in the offensive-defensive problem."[72] By that time, MAD advocates such as McNamara had come to regard damage-limiting capability as unable to contribute to deterrence, whether using offensive counterforce strikes or active and passive defenses. According to Lt. General Glenn Kent, one of McNamara's strategic analysts, the Defense Secretary had rejected defense in 1964, based on a key study which showed that it would be cost effective to limit damage only if our goal was to preserve no more that 70 percent of the population.[73] Cost effective in this case means that it would be cheaper to expand defense forces than for the potential opponent to expand his offensive forces. According to General Kent, McNamara believed that it must be cost effective to protect more than 90 percent of our population in order for damage-limiting work to make sense. However, in his 1969 reflections on his tenure in office, McNamara echoed Douhet: "It has been alleged that we are opposed to deploying a large-cycle ABM system because it would carry the heavy price tag of $40 billion. Let me make it very clear that the $40 billion is not the issue. If we could build and deploy a genuinely inpenetrable shield over the United States, we would be willing to spend not only $40 billion, but any reasonable multiple of that amount that was necessary."[74]

Robert McNamara and Hans Bethe's 1985 *Atlantic Monthly* article is as concise a summary of MAD doctrine and the role of defense as any in the literature. The soul of MAD is absolute rejection of military roles for nuclear weapons. The *Atlantic Monthly* article states simply: "All are saying directly or by implication, that nuclear weapons serve no military purpose whatsoever. They are not weapons. They are totally useless except to deter one's opponents from using his warheads."

The role of defense in a MAD world can be only one of two possibilities, what McNamara and Bethe call "Star Wars I"—an impenetrable shield, or "Star Wars II"—defense with retaliatory forces. Perfect defense is not possible technically, say the MAD theorists. If this were not so, they argue, defense would replace deterrence, not strengthen it. The fact that these theorists see no significant difference between militarily significant delivery systems like the MIRVed ICBM, and militarily ridiculous delivery systems like bombs hidden in Soviet diplomats' suitcases, underscores the total rejection of military significance for nuclear weapons. Defense of retaliatory assets, while acceptable, is rejected on the grounds that survivability for retaliatory forces may be more easily accomplished by other means such as launching those while under attack—a tactic non-MAD analysts regard as risky at best.

MAD strategists believe that defense for any comprehensive purpose is an implicit acceptance that nuclear warfighting can occur and is logical in some circumstances. McNamara and his colleagues fear that strategic defense means that nuclear weapons are militarily useful. Once this notion is accepted, the basic MAD precept of infinite offense must be rejected. Then, the Clausewitzian view of offensive and defensive roles comes to the fore. The surprise attack or first strike becomes the best strategy. Defense is relied upon to mop up the enemy's ragged response. According to MAD advocates, a large-scale defensive effort by either the United States or the Soviet Union would signal that nuclear warfighting, and particularly first-strike strategies, had been adopted over MAD.

Scientific Dispassion and the Strategic Debate

The entry of physicists into international politics and military strategy occurred on 16 July 1945. One might have expected that this would have marked a new era of rationality where the intellectual rigor and empirical exactitude of the laboratory would be transferred to international relations. Unfortunately, this has not been the case.

While Bernard Brodie defined the physicists' strategy in 1946, he also pointed out that the scientists were not approaching the problem from a particularly detached perspective: "It is satisfying intellectually to have some basis for appraising in terms of probability the random estimates which have been presented to the public. Some of these estimates, it must be said, though emanating from distinguished scientists, are not marked by the scientific discipline which is so rigorously observed in the laboratory; certainly they cannot be regarded as dispassionate."[75]

Some scientists are so committed to a certain strategic philosophy that they sacrifice not only technical rigor but also ethical behavior to advance their cause. This trend accelerated in the 1980s to the point where it threatened public faith in our nation's scientists and engineers.

When the Reagan administration began espousing what its critics called a "warfighting" strategy in the early 1980s, MAD adherents quickly reacted. Groups of scientists with names like

"The Physicians for Social Responsibility," and "The Union of Concerned Scientists (UCS)," went to work. The names of these organizations seem to have been chosen to imply that those who are not members are irresponsible and unconcerned. I've already addressed the levels of scorn such groups heaped upon civil defense advocates.

A second fundamental MAD dogma, the infeasibility of defense, has been challenged by the President's Strategic Defense Initiative. As an example of the emotional heat generated among physicists by the very suggestion that we pursue those, I compiled a set of pro-con papers on the SDI written by physicists.[76] To provide just one example of emotional appeals, personal attacks, sarcastic comments, and the like, the principal authors of the Union of Concerned Scientists' anti-SDI reports referred to an argument by Robert Jastrow, a pro-SDI scientist, in the following professional manner: "He has failed to notice that he is impaled on his own sword, blunt instrument though it may be."[77] Such a high density of non-technical arguments in short papers (10 or fewer pages) from technical experts is astounding. Although these curious arguments are concentrated on the part of strategic defense critics, they are by no means confined there. However, the fervor of MAD advocates has gone beyond mere emotion. I have chosen one example to illustrate my point—the question of how many orbital laser battle stations would be needed to counter the current Soviet ICBM inventory of some 1500 missiles.

I relate an example of scientific sleight-of-hand performed in the service of defeating the SDI. This example shows how far from scientific rigor the scientists have gone in pushing their strategic agenda. In March 1983, critics of the SDI were quick to seize on space-based lasers as the basis for President Reagan's Strategic Defense Initiative. Not surprisingly, these critics chose one of the least likely approaches for strategic defense. The Defensive Technologies Study (the 1983 study which formed the technical basis of the SDI) placed space-based lasers at a lower priority than most other defensive weapons concepts. Despite this well-known fact, or perhaps because of it, SDI critics chose space-based laser windmills to tilt against. In March 1984 the Union of Concerned Scientists published with much fanfare a report showing that 2400 space-based lasers of a type generally believed feasible would be needed to counter the *current* Soviet offensive arsenal.[78] (See figure 4.) The UCS report was authored by nine individuals—mostly physicists. Two of these, Richard Garwin and Hans Bethe, were members of JASON, a Defense advisory group. JASON had full access to the Defensive Technology Study reports and should have known that space-based lasers were not recommended.

The Department of Defense quickly pointed out that these laser calculations were wrong. Finding the 2400 number untenable, the UCS spokesman, Richard Garwin, said in open testimony before the Senate Armed Services Committee on 24 April 1984 that the correct number was 800.[79] In the September 1984 *Scientific American*, the UCS changed without comment its number to 300.[80] During this period, detailed computer calculations emerged from the Los Alamos and Livermore National Laboratories setting the correct number near 100.[81] In a series of increasingly abusive letters from Garwin to Gregory Canavan at Los Alamos, the UCS number slowly dropped, first to 142, then to 72.[82] This conclusion should have been the end of the incident, but it was not. In a series of public debates with me in 1985 and 1986 Garwin concocted a wide variety of calculations purporting to show that thousands of lasers would be needed.[83] Yet, Garwin's calculations are not for space-based lasers against the current Soviet threat, but against a totally new, hypothetical and strategically dubious Soviet threat—one that the Defensive Technologies study deemed unlikely for two decades or more.[84]

My purpose in reviewing this arcane debate is not to educate you on how many lasers are needed for an effective strategic defense system. Rather, the debate represents one skirmish in a much broader battle over the basis of our national strategy. That this debate is emotional is unarguable and probably to be expected; but the importance of the issues at stake reinforces the need for objective and ethical debate.

If a scientist errs because of insufficient knowledge, or even resorts to some data manipulation, that is not new or surprising. Yet, if results were presented which one knew to be wrong — that would be unethical. Figure 4 shows what Robert Jastrow calls the "Garwin Learning Curve," plotting the laser argument with time. This curve may be merely the result of

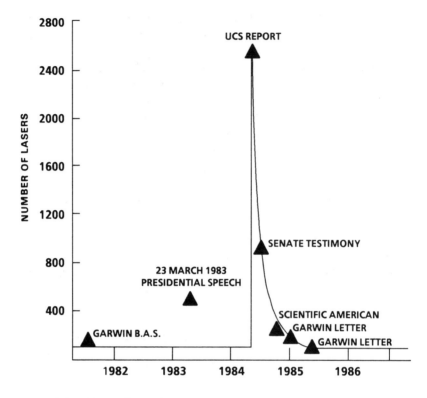

NOTE: ESTIMATES ARE FOR SAME TYPE OFFENSIVE FORCE AND
       SAME TYPE DEFENSIVE SATELLITE

Source: Data courtesy of Dr. Robert Jastrow, Dartmouth College.

Figure 4. History of Estimates of Union of Concerned Scientists on Number of Lasers Required for Strategic Defense. Shown are the published estimates of the Union of Concerned Scientists on the number of laser satellites needed to defend against the current Soviet ICBM force. Also plotted are the accepted results of Department of Defense experts.

slow correction of an optimistic calculation. But I draw your attention to a calculation Garwin made in 1981 of a similar problem.[85] Although the calculation and parameters are slightly different than the 1984-85 debate, I note that the results agree with the long-standing DOD values close to 100, and not the UCS numbers. Thus, Garwin and his colleagues grossly miscalculated, to say the least. When their mistakes were pointed out to them, their reaction was curious: rather than welcoming the improved data in a genuine spirit of scientific questing for accuracy, these critics responded with vicious personal attacks. For example, Garwin sent letters threatening legal action to both national laboratories, complaining about those who pointed out his errors.[86]

The scientific advocates frequently assert that MAD is not a theory, but a "fact of life,"[87] a sort of physical law. However, as Albert Wohlstetter pointed out, scientists "don't sign agreements to abide by the third law of thermodynamics."[88]

From MAD to a Non-Deterrent Approach: Disarmament

Pacifist approaches to the nuclear problem have a history as long as that of the weapon. Albert Einstein, who may have borne some remorse over his role in persuading President Roosevelt to start the atomic bomb project, became an eloquent and persuasive advocate of world government. Although the physicists who developed the atomic bomb made repeated efforts to place atomic energy under international control as early as 1943[89] and founded the *Bulletin of the Atomic Scientists* in the fall of 1945, Einstein was the main spokesperson after the war. He led the way not only for international control of atomic energy, but for a world government maintaining its power through sole possession of nuclear weapons. In 1946 Einstein wrote:

> The available weapons of destruction are of a kind such that no place on Earth is safeguarded against sudden total destruction. The only hope for protection lies in securing the peace in a supranational way. A world government must be created which is able to solve conflicts between nations by judicial decision. This government must be

based on a clear-cut constitution which is approved by the governments and nations and which gives it sole disposition of offensive weapons.[90]

Einstein's desire for world government began long before the atomic bomb, but the existence of an "infinite" weapon gave his case urgency. Einstein and other scientists believed that tyranny from a world government was preferable to the end of the world.[91] As one of his final efforts, Einstein teamed up with Bertrand Russell, the renowned British humanist and socialist. Out of these efforts the "Pugwash Conferences" grew. These brought together scientists from both sides of the East-West dispute to work out differences, with the goal of eliminating nuclear weapons. The first Pugwash Conference was in 1957. These meetings continue, but have turned into meetings of largely left-leaning Western scientists and Soviet disinformation artists from the USA-Canada Institute in Moscow.[92]

Bertrand Russell became notorious with several extreme positions he held. Although he had made it clear he did not seek unilateral disarmament, he thought it preferable to continuing with a MAD deterrent.[93] This "better red than dead" view has always been popular in Europe, but never caught on in the United States. Russell was also an early proponent of "We're as bad as you" overtures to the Soviet Union.[94] The logic proceeds from an idea that public awareness that "we" are as bad as "they" could lead to more acceptance of solutions which let them win. From this perspective, nationalism is less likely to stand in the way of nuclear disarmament.

In addition to assaults from the intellectual and scientific left, some national security experts also questioned deterrence theory (MAD or otherwise).[95] These analysts began to view deterrence as part of the problem. They rejected both the "chicken" model and the assumption that the players were rational. Among their observations:

● States would rather keep what they've got than acquire new assets.

● States place different values on items of "national interest." It is not possible to play chicken when it's clear one side is less interested.

• States behave far more moderately than deterrence theory predicts. They don't go to the brink very often.

• Deterrence theory exaggerates the costs of backing down. Rewards as well as punishment play a role in deterrence.

• Deterrence theory ignores politics. What are the conflicts really about?

The net result of the intellectual and scientific attack on MAD deterrence was to lessen the perceived threat from the Soviet Union in the late 1970s. Many believed that international problems were the fault of deterrence as much as they stemmed from unacceptable Soviet behavior. The thought that our problems with the Soviets would go away if the weapons went away gained strength from these diverse arguments.

In the early 1980s the perceived need to deter the Soviet Union was lessening and the perception of a sure nuclear Armageddon mounting. Morality concerns cropped up and were manifested in the US Roman Catholic bishops' grappling with the morality of deterrence. Catholic dogma has always contained elements of conflicting views. On one hand the Church supports "just wars" to counter evil (jus ad bellum). On the other hand, some elements of the Church have always adopted a strictly pacifist view. Generally, the just war tradition has been dominant. But the morality of deterrence, if it involved the end of the world and mass death of millions of innocent people (by the hand of man, not God), was different. After much discussion and soul-searching, the US Catholic bishops cautiously condemned strategies involving the death of innocent people. The apocalyptic views of the Union of Concerned Scientists and the Physicians for Social Responsibility played an important role in those deliberations.[96]

Since 1983 and the Catholic Bishops' Pastoral Letter on War and Peace, other more radical moral conclusions have emerged. The United Methodist bishops—also lobbied by people like Carl Sagan—strongly condemned MAD deterrence.[97]

In the mid–1980s, others also rejected MAD deterrence as immoral and dangerous. Inherent in views like those of Jonathan Schell and Freeman Dyson is the finite possibility of the end of the world.[98] Since deterrence must have a finite possibility of nuclear war to be credible, the possibility of an infinitely bad outcome (everyone dead) cannot be balanced by the fact that the possibility of war happening is only "small."

A coalition of religious activists and the American left rejects deterrence. These groups look to scientists to reinforce the end-of-the-world view. This beyond-MAD approach has the following precepts:

● The continued existence of nuclear weapons will ultimately mean the end of the world. Since it can happen tomorrow, the problem is urgent today.

● MAD, or any other form of deterrence which allows nuclear weapons, is immoral and dangerous.

● Nothing is more important than survival. Radical solutions such as world government and unilateral disarmament should not be rejected.

● The US Government, because it possesses nuclear weapons, is as morally bankrupt as the Soviet Union. Since the US Government is accessible, it is appropriate to attack it as a co-conspirator. It helps to point out all of the bad things the US Government is doing.

2. RETALIATION-BASED NUCLEAR DETERRENCE

The second deterrent strategy emerged from traditional military wisdom. Since nations are run by politicians and armies led by soldiers, the logic of deterrence must be the logic of these leaders, not the logic of physicists and academics. Our best-known Prussian strategists defined this theory of deterrence in terms with meaning to politicians and soldiers:

> Combat is the only effective force in war; its aim is to destroy the enemy's forces as a means to a further end. That holds good even if no actual fighting occurs, because the outcome rests on the assumption that if it comes to fighting, the enemy would be destroyed. It follows that the destruction of the enemy's force underlies all military actions; all plans are ultimately based on it like an arch on its abutment. Consequently all action is undertaken in the belief that if the ultimate test of arms should actually occur the outcome would be *favorable*.
>
> General Karl von Clausewitz
> 1818

A famous American general, George Patton, translated this concept in 1943 into a short form easily understood by our leaders and people: "No dumb bastard ever won a war by going out and dying for his country. He won it by making some other dumb bastard die for his country."

When children become teenagers they develop annoying rejoinders to instructions: "But you don't follow your own rules!" The response: "Do what I say, not what I do!" may serve for teenagers, but not for national strategic policy. We speak of MAD but follow General Clausewitz—or at least General Patton. Every president since Harry Truman has talked about the horror of nuclear war. Each has spoken of blasted cities, of mass death, and of the end of the world. But every one has signed directives to the troops that are much different.

Strategic targets are and have always been the other nation's troops and the means of supporting them—not the fabric of enemy society. In this chapter I will discuss how US nuclear strategy has evolved and what it means.

The Way We Are: Nuclear Warfighting

Since the first caveman heaved a rock at the guy in the next cave, mankind has fought wars for just two reasons: banditry and ideology. The human desire to get what others have—which I define as banditry—permeates history. From the ancient Celtic legend of the Cattle Raid of Cuailnge to Hitler's quest for *"Lebensraum,"* greed has motivated armed action. MAD theory assumes that it is the sole reason for war. Since nuclear war would always leave the "victor" in worse shape, regardless of his war gains, MAD holds that no nation could rationally entertain the possibility of nuclear war. If the bandit nation is destroyed there will be no one to enjoy the spoils. But wars also arise from clashes of ideas. Our problem has been how to deter not just bandits, but also an Islamic jihad, a Christian crusade, or a Marxist revolution.

Ideological wars have always been with us. But 19th century technology and ideology made entire societies full participants in the fray. Napoleon brought us modern war. He showed that an entire people could be mobilized for war, the first European to do so. His war was total war—the citizen soldier supported by the entire society of a nation in a quest for a new world order. General von Clausewitz understood this total war as no one has before or since. In Clausewitz's *On War* I find the seeds of deterrence in the second half of the 20th century—and not in the nuclear-fused sand at Trinity Site, New Mexico.[1]

Clausewitz presented his ideas in a form familiar to Marxists—the dialectic. He first related theory in pure form and then contrasted it with reality. Out of contrast came new wisdom. He began *On War* with a discussion of war in its pure form. Pure war persuades the enemy through force. In Clausewitz's words, "If the enemy is to be coerced you must put him in a situation that is even more unpleasant than the sacrifice you call on him to make.'' Clausewitz then told us how to do this: "If you are to force the enemy, by making war on him to do your bidding, you must either make him literally defenseless or at least put him in a position that makes this danger probable. It follows that to overcome the enemy, or disarm him—call it what you will—must always be the aim of war.''[2]

Clausewitz was quick to point out that this approach to war was theoretical. Many factors modify the real world—politics, economics, and emotions, to name a few. But Clausewitz didn't dismiss pure war entirely:

> Would this ever be the case in practice? Yes, it would if: (a) war was a wholly isolated act, occurring suddenly and not produced by previous events in the polemical world; (b) it consisted of a single decisive act or a set of simultaneous ones; (c) the decision achieved was complete and perfect in itself, uninfluenced by any previous estimate of the political situation it would bring about.[3]

I showed in chapter 1 how nuclear weapons make General Douhet's counter-society tactics possible. These key weapons also make General Clausewitz's pure-form war plausible.

What have the nuclear-armed nations made of these classical strategies? As I will show in chapter 4, the Soviet Union has fully embraced Clausewitz.[4] To be sure, the United States hasn't ignored Clausewitzian theory either. We have taken parts of it, combining other ideas to produce a remarkably consistent strategy—one we have not altered since World War II.

While the United States flirts with MAD rhetoric, it plans for war based on Clausewitz's ideas. To that strategy US theorists have added Douhet's tactics. Nuclear weapons have been combined with fast delivery systems, and this combination makes a decisive war possible. The chance of decisive Western victory has been used to coerce the Soviet Union into accepting Western goals, goals which may be as simple as refraining from actions which risk nuclear war. Douhet told us that we must rely solely on offensive forces as our instrument. I propose the following as true precepts of US deterrence:

- We must prepare for a single massive nuclear exchange with the Soviet Union.

- Our target is the armed might of the Soviet Union, not its people.

- Our primary tool is our strategic offensive nuclear force.

US strategic rhetoric swings between the reality of Clausewitz and Douhet and the MAD vision of the physicists. Since 1945 at least two full cycles have run their course. During each, stated US policy slowly drifted toward MAD, but real nuclear strategy did not follow. When the inconsistency between action strategy and stated policy became great enough, arcane strategic debates became public.

The first rhetorical cycle peaked in the late 1950s. Secretary of State John Foster Dulles triggered the public debate with his so-called "new look" massive retaliation rhetoric in 1954.[5] Massive retaliation was, in fact, nothing more than US intent to rely on nuclear might to deter war. The public, however, came to understand that Soviet cities were to be held hostage to Soviet good behavior. Critics of massive retaliation—among them Henry Kissinger[6] and Army Chief of Staff General Maxwell D. Taylor[7]—developed a counter strategy, "Flexible Response." The critics' strategy still relied on nuclear weapons. But Flexible Response made explicit provision, at least in theory, for less than all-out war and even non-nuclear war. When the Kennedy administration took office in 1961, it wasted no time in making Flexible Response official strategy.

The second rhetorical cycle has been, perhaps justifiably so, laid at the doorstep of Robert McNamara, Secretary of Defense in the Kennedy administration, who became preoccupied with nuclear forces designed to commit "Assured Destruction"—the guaranteed devastation of an enemy's society. McNamara's quest was to maintain a survivable nuclear force sufficient for committing assured destruction. This basis for deterrence became his dominant concern.[8] Chapter 1 outlines this strategy—now known as MAD.

Throughout the 1970s, US official pronouncements rejected assured destruction, or MAD, as our deterrent basis. The United States preferred what I can only call a nuclear warfighting strategy. The Nixon administration called it "sufficiency,"[9] and the Carter administration called it "countervailing strategy."[10]

In reality, the differences were of rhetoric alone. Since 1945 the United States has maintained a warfighting nuclear deterrent strategy. The term "warfighting" is, unfortunately, a loaded word. But as used in this chapter, "warfighting" means that the United States deters war by maintaining nuclear offensive forces sufficient to beat an aggressor, even if struck first.

US Warfighting Strategy Since World War II

To recognize the truth, one must often step outside the problem. The description of US strategy closest to the mark is an attack on it by a Soviet propagandist, Henry Trofimenko: "Instead of an evolution of strategy, we see only semantic convolutions: 'sufficiency,' 'rough parity,' 'approximate parity,' 'essential equivalence,' and 'countervailing strategy.' All of these terms, as a matter of fact, are employed as guises for one and the same strategy of flexible response."[11]

Trofimenko is right; the United States has not changed its action strategy since World War II. To that list I also add "massive retaliation" and "assured destruction."

In support of my contention I need look no further than comments by senior military officials. For example, General David Jones, then Chairman of the Joint Chiefs of Staff, testified on this subject before Congress on 24 July 1979. When asked about MAD he said:

> I do not subscribe to the idea that we ever had it [MAD] as our basic strategy. I have been involved with strategic forces since the early 1950s. We have always targeted military targets. There has been a lot of discussion, when I was out in the field, [and] in Washington you would hear a lot of rhetoric about different strategies. We followed orders, but basically, the strategy stayed the same in implementation of targeting.[12]

The United States and Britain believed they could win World War II by strategic bombing. Britain devoted 50 percent of its war production to the Royal Air Force and the United States spent 35 percent of its war effort on the Air Corps.[13]

World War II targets were the enemy's means of waging war—his industrial and transportation systems. But these targets were in urban areas. Strategic bombing thus became associated with large-scale civilian destruction—if only as a by-product of attacks on military targets. The atomic bomb was 1000 times more powerful than conventional bombs, but it didn't change the strategy, it only made it more efficient. With atomic bombs, a single bomber could do the job of hundreds.

The atomic attack on Hiroshima was a case in point. The city contained several important military targets—war-supporting industries on its outskirts and a key bridge at its heart.[14] The bridge was the chosen target and the atomic bomb dispatched it unambiguously. But the industries on Hiroshima's periphery were almost undamaged.[15] The bomb had greatly increased the mass destruction side effects, but was a more modest advance as a military weapon. My calculation of military effectiveness at the end of the introduction shows that the atomic bomber was more effective than a conventional bomber—but not by the great factor of increase in explosive power of the bomb. A single conventional bomber could have destroyed the bridge just as well as the plane with the atomic bomb.

In the 1940s and early 1950s US bombing ideas remained those of World War II.[16] There were three target classes:

1. War-supporting industries such as aircraft production facilities.

2. Transportation links and points such as roads and rail centers.

3. Military forces such as Soviet air bases.

What changed in the mid-1950s to alter US strategic rhetoric? The answer is simple—the election of Republicans and the development of hydrogen bombs.

In 1952 Eisenhower swept the Republicans into office on a platform of fiscal responsibility, in particular pledging massive defense cuts. Secretary of State Dulles's "New Look" was the result. Far from a fundamental change in strategic doctrine, it was an economy move, placing basic national security squarely with our strategic nuclear forces. The Air Force became first in importance, the Army received drastic cuts, the Navy less drastic ones.[17]

Hydrogen bombs—so-called because they derive some of their energy from hydrogen fusion and fusion-induced nuclear fission—represent a 1000-fold increase in destructive power over atomic fission bombs. This is as big an increase as atomic bombs over conventional weapons. The scientific community plunged into the political fray over whether we needed such a weapon.[18] By entering this public debate the scientists politically lost their impartiality. Robert Oppenheimer and other left-of-center physicists opposed what they viewed as wanton destructiveness unjustified by military requirements. If the United States already had a hammer and only wanted to kill flies, a steam-driven sledge suggested excess. Moreover, it was argued, US restraint in developing the hydrogen bomb might lead the Soviet Union to similar restraint.

Arrayed against Robert Oppenheimer were the Air Force and its scientific allies, most notably Edward Teller, who argued for the hydrogen bomb out of technological determinism. Because it could be done, the Soviets would do it, and therefore the United States must have it first. Oppenheimer's military sufficiency arguments were right—today's US strategic arsenal has few weapons much larger than 1950s fission bombs. Teller was also right—the Soviet Union was already well on its way to a hydrogen bomb regardless of US actions.[19]

The hydrogen bomb, a million times more powerful than a World War II conventional bomb, entered our inventory in the mid-1950s. From a military standpoint the extra power offered few dividends. Yet it multiplied potential civilian deaths many times over. Since early hydrogen bombs were only efficient as killers of people, the public came to believe that the sole purpose of nuclear forces was mass civilian death. Massive retaliation came to mean mass destruction. Objections to the mass destruction perception came from two quarters—intellectual analysis and interservice rivalry.

The most formidable was the second: interservice rivalry. After the Korean War the Army demobilized. The frugally-minded Eisenhower administration accelerated this process. By the mid-1950s the Army had only 10 percent of the defense budget share—less than one-fifth the Air Force portion. The reason was Air Force nuclear weapons. The Army response was to get a piece of the mission. The vehicle was to be a new doctrine, flexible response, as an alternative to massive retaliation.[20]

The Army Chief of Staff from 1955 to 1959, General Maxwell D. Taylor, was an advocate of flexible response. He wasted no time after his retirement in 1959 in pressing his views. In his book, *The Uncertain Trumpet*,[21] he said of flexible response:

> It is just as necessary to deter or win quickly a limited war as to deter general war. Otherwise, the limited war which cannot be won quickly may result in piecemeal attrition or involvement in an expanding conflict which may grow into the general war we all want to avoid.[22]

General Taylor didn't mince words. Flexible response was a warfighting strategy which "would restore warfare to its historic justification as a means to create a better world upon the successful conclusion of hostilities."[23] Although he acknowledged that the conflict between flexible response and massive retaliation had "theological" overtones,[24] he also believed that the gulf could be bridged. He noted an article by massive retaliation's originator, John Foster Dulles, citing a need for low-yield battlefield nuclear weapons.[25] Dulles' famous 1954 massive retaliation speech did not mention attacks on civilians as the basis of deterrence. Nor can I find any such official statement in the late 1950s to this effect. The view that MAD grew out of massive retaliation appears insupportable.

Flexible response doctrine focused on three military capabilities. Not surprisingly, General Taylor identified these as Army responsibilities:[26]

1. Strategic Defense in the form of the nuclear-armed *Army* Nike Zeus as an ABM against the emerging Soviet ICBM threat. The General made it clear that Nike Zeus supported US retaliatory forces, not population defense, "It is the only system currently under development which will be capable of defending our retaliatory forces ... against ballistic missiles."[27]

2. Battlefield nuclear weapons for a ground nuclear conflict. Sufficient ground forces were needed to defeat and occupy enemy territory.

3. Intermediate-range nuclear armed ballistic missile forces.

What General Taylor laid out in strategic theory, his protégé, Lieutenant General James Gavin, expanded in tactical form. His 1959 book, *War and Peace in the Space Age*, advocated an air- and, eventually, space-mobile army.[28] To fight on a nuclear battlefield, forces were to be extremely decentralized and backed up with nuclear-armed missiles.

I especially note two of General Gavin's ideas. He was the first to emphasize the decisive role of space. Following the analysis at the end of the Introduction I call attention to Gavin's foresight on this subject: "Of one thing we may be sure, the nation that first achieves the control of outer space will control the destiny of the human race."[29]

General Gavin also recognized that nuclear strategy was becoming partisan. He identified massive retaliation with Republican conservatives and flexible response with Democratic liberals. From the 1950s on, nuclear strategy took on partisan political overtones—to the detriment of a coherent US policy. A number of strategic thinkers provided intellectual underpinning for flexible response, in particularly Paul Nitze, Henry Kissinger, and Albert Wohlstetter.[30]

Paul Nitze's analyses were seminal and direct. His 1956 *Foreign Affairs* article separated US declaratory policy—massive retaliation or assured destruction at the time—from US *action* policy, which Nitze called "graduated deterrence."[31] He recognized that winning a nuclear war in the World War II sense is impossible. Even the victor would not be better off than if the war hadn't occurred. But a nation could "win" a nuclear war in postwar comparisons between the victor and the vanquished. The side that would win in this comparison would have the strongest deterrent.

Nitze argued that the United States could best meet this goal by carefully considering only military objectives, and that deterrence based on destroying industrial and population centers was to be avoided. He identified air superiority as the single most important objective: "Once he has gained control of the intercontinental air space, then his enemy's entire country, including cities, industries, means of communications and remaining military capabilities will be open to attack.'' He hit the nail on the head, since ICBMs made air space into aerospace. Nitze and Gavin said the same thing—control space and you control the world.

Henry Kissinger's 1957 book, *Nuclear Weapons and Foreign Policy*, expanded on flexible response in exhaustive, if not exhausting, detail.[32] Kissinger integrated nuclear weapons into a coherent global strategy for the West, designing an approach based on realistic appraisals of Soviet intentions, strengths and weaknesses.

Henry Kissinger's greatest contribution was his understanding of historical American attitudes. For the United States, superior resources and technology have always been more important than a superior strategy. Soviet strategy, he argued, was also consistent since at least the 1920s. To be sure, it was also Marxist and, from a US perspective, evil. Kissinger discussed the popular view of massive retaliation as a threat to annihilate Soviet society, considering such a response to Soviet foreign transgressions not as a strategy, but as a refusal to have one.

Dr. Kissinger especially decried the threat of all-out war as our *only* response to Soviet aggression. This approach, he said, would only encourage the Soviet Union to engage in all sorts of aggression, as long as they stopped short of actions which the United States felt worth total war. The Korean War was an example of just such limited aggression. Kissinger proposed United States responses the American people might consider actually using, proclaiming, in his words, that ''deterrence is greatest when military strength is coupled with the willingness to employ it.''[33] In short, the United States must be ready to fight limited wars—be they between secondary powers, superpowers or both. However sensible these views were to grand nuclear strategy, they contained the seeds of the Vietnam war.

Flexible response doctrine was the first explicit recognition that all-out nuclear war strategies could decouple US security from that of Western Europe. Limited attacks were and still are the most likely Soviet threats to Europe, and such attacks call for limited responses. Kissinger believed that Europe would accept its fair share of the Western defense burden if every move did not risk ultimate catastrophe. He identified the United States as an "island" power similar to 19th-century Britain. US objectives should be, like Britain's before, to prevent hegemony in Europe and Asia—not to bring on a final battle which the West might well lose. To this end Kissinger advocated limited nuclear war options. The European powers themselves might provide or at least control the nuclear weapons.

The final contribution of the 1950s, and the most lasting one, grew out of Soviet and not US warfighting strategies. Soviet ballistic missiles—capable of striking US nuclear forces—raise the specter of a devastating Soviet first strike, one which could virtually wipe out Western abilities to effectively retaliate.

Albert Wohlstetter's 1959 *Foreign Affairs* article laid the groundwork for almost every strategic analysis since.[34] The scenario began with a Soviet strike against US nuclear forces. The issue was whether the United States would preserve sufficient nuclear forces to strike back in a militarily effective way. In short, do we have enough survivable nuclear weapons to win the war even if ours is a second strike?

President Kennedy took office in 1961, owing his victory in part to a largely imaginary "missile gap." The Soviet Union was, incorrectly, thought to have enough ICBMs to remove an effective US military retaliation. The Kennedy administration made flexible response its official policy. Robert McNamara's 16 June 1962 speech in Ann Arbor, Michigan made US action policy match declared policy.

> The United States has come to the conclusion that to the extent feasible, basic military strategy in a possible general nuclear war should be approached in much the same way that more conventional military operations have been in the past. That is to say, principal military objectives, in the event of nuclear war stemming from a major attack on the Alliance, should be the destruction of the enemy's military forces, not of his civilian population.[35]

As I showed earlier, Robert McNamara gradually shifted to a MAD declaratory strategy. Not surprisingly, our military forces and targeting policy stayed attuned to warfighting. Military targets and not people have always been programmed in the weapon computers. Figure 5 shows US strategic forces during

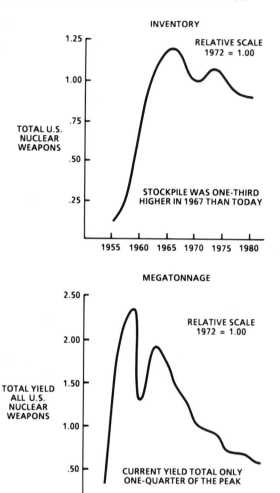

Source: DOD testimony in hearings before the Committee on Armed Services, US Senate, 98th Congress, 2d session, February 1, 1984 (Washington, DC: US Government Printing Office, 1984), p. 122.

Figure 5. Status of US Nuclear Weapon Stockpile. Note the 25% decrease in warheads and 25% decrease in megatonnage.

this period, both in total numbers of weapons and megatonnage. Throughout the 1960s and 1970s—periods of great rhetorical swings in strategic policy—nuclear forces only evolved slowly. Warhead numbers first stabilized and then went down. More significantly, total megatonnage decreased greatly. Our nuclear forces became more precise and ready for warfighting. How could this have happened—particularly in the late 1960s when MAD was hammered into public consciousness and presidential directives? Meanwhile, Robert McNamara and other politicos emphasized number of Soviets killed as the basis of deterrence. By MAD logic, the United States should have moved toward a *greatly* reduced number of warheads with greatly *increased* individual destructiveness. A handful of multi-megaton city-busters would have done the trick. The answer lies in strategic force justifications of US planners.

Morton Halperin, a senior strategic planner from the Johnson and Nixon administrations, provided some clues.[36] The Department of Defense pulled a "fast one." Strategic planners interpreted assured destruction requirements in such a way to actually support a warfighting force structure. As I noted earlier in this chapter, General David Jones implied that US strategic targeting planners ignored assured destruction.

McNamara's assured destruction doctrine required destroying 25 percent of the Soviet population. As I discussed earlier, McNamara now thought 1000-2000 warheads could do it. How, then, did the DOD ever justify the 10,000 warheads they had in the late 1960s?

First, Morton Halperin answered, the Department of Defense had to plan for a "worse-than-possible" first-strike threat. That preparation would mean that warhead requirements would have to be doubled, up to about 4000. But, it was felt, more would be needed. What if the Soviets made useless (destroyed or damaged) one or more legs of the Triad? The answer would be to make each leg independently able to assure destruction. With three legs, that is, bombers, land-based missiles, and sea-based missiles, I count another factor of three! Alas, the United States needed about 12,000 warheads to assure destruction. It all adds up. The strategic planners used assured destruction requirements to justify a warfighting deterrent. No policy maker in Washington must ever have checked to see where warheads were really aimed.

The 1970s saw a second retreat from MAD rhetoric. Two factors contributed. First, the imaginary "missile gap" of the 1950s became a reality in the 1970s. A disarming Soviet missile strike against US retaliatory forces was possible. Second, arms control became a central element in US national security. The United States pursued arms control based on a MAD strategic doctrine while its force structure was warfighting. The mismatch between arms control and military strategies was, and remains, a serious threat to our national security.

In 1970 President Nixon asked some questions:

> Should a President, in the event of a nuclear attack, be left with the single option of ordering the mass destruction of enemy civilians, in the face of the certainty that it would be followed by the mass slaughter of Americans? Should the concept of assured destruction be narrowly defined and should it be the only measure of our ability to deter the variety of threats we face?[37]

Secretary of Defense James Schlesinger gave President Nixon an answer in 1974.[38] In that year's Defense Posture Statement he defined what the Nixon and Ford administrations meant by "strategic sufficiency," stating that the United States must have a variety of options short of destroying enemy cities. Schlesinger specifically pointed out that appropriate nuclear targets were more than the cities and missile silos discussed in the past—they also included, and might even be dominated, by such others as airfields and other military installations. Some experts point out that a true flexible response targeting doctrine did not exist prior to the 1974 strategic directives.[39] It may be that, prior to 1974, the strategic planners no more had real limited plans than they had assured destruction targeting. At the least there were no formal directives mandating such limited options.

Soviet power grew throughout the 1970s—to the point of actual Soviet superiority in the late years of that decade. As the saying goes, nothing focuses the mind like the imminent prospect of one's own hanging. So it was with US strategic thinkers. The most pessimistic was Colin Gray, author of several articles on this topic.[40] He resurfaced the ancient concept of military victory as the basis of national strategy, pointing out in 1979 that nuclear war is not impossible merely because it is horrible. "Deterrence must work within the enemy's mind," he said. Gray continued, "Deterrence cannot deter unless we know what influences that mind. Soviet leaders just might perceive the world differently." Gray stressed that Soviet leaders fear defeat—not damage. They, not US academics, define what defeat is. To deter war, he insisted, the United States must present the Soviet Union with the likelihood of Soviet defeat—in short, US victory. In his words, "One of the essential tasks of the American defense community is to help ensure that in moments of acute crisis the Soviet general staff cannot brief the Politburo with a plausible theory of military victory."[41]

Gray and others had an impact. Secretary of Defense Harold Brown announced the "countervailing strategy" in 1979: "We must have forces, contingency plans and command and control capabilities that will convince the Soviet leadership that no war and no course of aggression by them that led to the use of nuclear weapons—on any scale of attack and at any stage of conflict—could lead to victory, however they may define victory."[42]

The United States explicitly recognized some long-held Soviet perceptions. As I will discuss, the Soviet Union plans for prolonged nuclear war. The Soviets believe that military forces and not economic capacity should be initial targets, and that survival of the regime is the highest priority. Finally, they insist on the possibility of victory in nuclear war. To deter them, the United States must target the things valued most, Soviet military and political leadership, Soviet command and control, conventional and nuclear forces, and the means to sustain war.[43]

To the Reagan administration fell the task of building the forces needed. These forces included offensive systems—the MX, heavy ICBM, and the submarine-launched D-5 missile. These are forces accurate enough to dig out hardened and protected Soviet forces, control mechanisms, and leadership. The United States also added forces, such as cruise missiles, which are flexible and able to locate mobile armed might and penetrate Soviet defenses to destroy it. In short, the United States sought the forces needed to hit the Soviet Army hard. This might be technically feasible, but I believe it is politically impossible.

Although the focus of my discussion is not arms control, we cannot ignore it either. For, as I defined national strategy earlier, it shares equal importance with both offensive and defensive forces. Arms control entered the US strategic arsenal in the late 1960s, and the SALT I and ABM Treaties of 1972 were its first significant results. I join many experts who believe that arms control, as practiced, has weakened US security. The problem is MAD. Since our strategy has been and remains military and retaliation-based, the gap between idealism and this reality is dangerous. This gap was the second source of critical strategic thought in the 1970s.

Fred Ikle's 1973 *Foreign Affairs* article was among the first to focus on the arms control-strategy disconnect.[44] Arms control had been designed to preserve mutual destruction and halt the nuclear buildup. Ikle identified arms control's dogma as:

- Nuclear forces have the sole purpose of retaliation.
- Retaliation must be swift and massive.
- Retaliation must kill some significant fraction of the Soviet people.

Ikle challenged these with two theses:

1. War can occur through irrationality; however, MAD assumes rationality.
2. MAD is immoral.

His criticisms are eloquent and compelling, although dogmatic in their own way:

> What a sad irony that the nations that had to fight Hitler to his last bunker should now rely on an interlock of their military postures, making survival depend on the rationality of all future leaders in all major nuclear powers.
>
> Tomas de Torquemada, who burned 10,000 heretics at the stake, could claim principles more humane than our military strategy; for his tribunals found all of his victims guilty of having knowingly committed mortal sin.[45]

Paul Nitze considered arms control from a quantitative basis.[46] He looked at a host of strategic parameters: number of launchers, number of nuclear warheads, equivalent megatonnage, and counter-military potential (read this as warfighting.) In the 1970s and 1980s, the Soviet Union had built advantages in most of these measures, and arms control only made matters worse. Ambassador Nitze introduced the important concept of "nuclear blackmail." He believed an unacceptable dilemma might arise if the United States did not have a credible nuclear warfighting strategy:

> The current question is whether a future US President should be left with only the option of deciding within minutes, or at most within two or three hours, to retaliate after a counterforce attack in a manner certain to result not only in the defeat of the United States, but in wholly disproportionate and truly irremediable destruction to the American people.[47]

I have reviewed the cycles of rhetoric and strategic doctrine. US strategy has evolved slowly and has not always been consistent with stated positions. MAD calculates deterrence in Soviet deaths, but our real strategy measures it much differently.

Exchange Calculations and Strategic Stability

When the United States had nuclear weapons and the Soviets didn't, deterrence was easy to measure. We had an absolutely stable deterrent. You could measure it by all parameters—megatons, industrial destruction, military victory—take your pick. The United States would win. Out of this potential for victory we had a more stable deterrent than what has since developed.

Before I discuss some mathematics, let me define some basic concepts. The most important is *Crisis Stability*. It measures the pressures during an international crisis which either encourage or discourage nuclear weapons use. To see how these considerations work, suppose the Soviet Union invaded a small country tomorrow morning. Some factors would move the United States toward a military response—desire to deny Soviet gain, empathy for the victims, US public opinion, and so forth. Other considerations would argue for restraint—fear of nuclear war, the possibility of military defeat, domestic politics as examples. A strategic analyst tries to list these factors, or "quantify" them, by assigning numbers according to their importance. One way to quantify this problem is the decision matrix I described in chapter 1. From these numbers the analyst makes predictions. Out of this process, its enthusiasts believe, we can learn how to lessen the possibility of nuclear war.

I point out two special aspects of crisis stability.[48] Some considerations will *tempt* a country to strike—namely the possibility of winning the war by getting in the first blows. Other factors will *pressure* a nuclear strike—the very real worry that the other guy will get in his hits first. Proper analysis must deal with both temptations and pressures during international crises.

What is strategic analysis, you might ask, since everybody seems to talk about it, experts get paid a lot for doing it, but yet nobody seems to be able to define the term? The best description that I know of is that strategic analysis is the answer to the question: "What is the big picture?" It is, I will add, a concept like "system engineering."

Strategic analysis has taken one of three forms: theoretical comparisons, war gaming, and practical estimates.[49] I will discuss each in turn.

Theoretical Comparisons

The simplest way to compare the superpowers' nuclear potential is to look at "static" measures. By static I mean how much of something each side has before a war. For example, I might count up all of the nuclear warheads each side has as one static measure of their relative power. Nitze compared various static measures of the two superpowers in the late 1970s.[50] In figure 6 I show recent trends in some key measures because they show the long-term increase in Soviet capability. Static measures have been the basis of most arms control negotiations. These various measures are:

- Total Megatonnage. To get this measure one adds the total explosive power of each side's nuclear arsenal. Total megatonnage is a good measure of assured destruction potential.[51] In the introduction I pointed out that radioactive fallout would produce the majority of deaths in an unprotected population. Megatons exploded

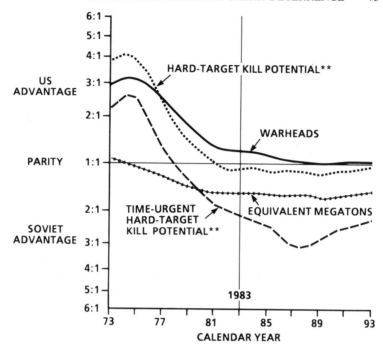

* TOTAL ACTIVE INVENTORY (INCLUDES FB-111 AND BACKFIRE)
** CALCULATIONS ARE BASED ON POTENTIAL AGAINST IDENTICAL HARDNESS TARGETS

Source: Report of the Secretary of Defense to Congress, February 1, 1984 (Washington, DC: US Government Printing Office, 1984), p. 434, in Hearings before the Committee on Armed Services, US Senate, February 1, 1987.

Figure 6. Strategic Forces* Pre-Attack Static Ratio Comparison.
Shown are ratios between US and Soviet forces in hard-target kill potential, warheads, equivalent megatons, and time-urgent, hard-target kill potential (first-strike accurate warheads loaded on ICBMs).

over cities directly translate into fallout levels. In the 1950s this was the preferred measure of relative strength.[52]

- Ballistic Missile *Throw Weight*. Since bigger missiles can deliver more bombs, its useful to know the weight in pounds that one side can "throw" with its missiles. Paul Nitze said this measure was the key to city-busting potential or "countervalue" targeting.[53] Civil defense is one reason why this is a good measure. To destroy a defended urban population one must destroy the city with the nuclear blast. Throw weight tells us both how many bombs an enemy can have and how big an area can be knocked down.

In the early 1970s Soviet bombs were large and inefficient. A Soviet bomb of the same megatonnage weighed much more than its US counterpart. For this reason the Soviet Union developed very large booster rockets. The 1970s' arms control agreements allowed the Soviets to keep a huge throw weight advantage. As Soviet technology improved—a fact the arms controllers should have foreseen—the Soviet Union translated that into advantages in total megatonnage and other measures. In the mid-1980s, the Soviet Union had a total throw weight of 5.4 million kilograms— the weight of a naval destroyer! (The United States has a total throw weight of 1.9 million kilograms.[54]) This Soviet advantage— allowed by arms control—has made it "tricky," to say the least, to get them to agree to equitable agreements. To preserve arms control possibilities some have sought long and hard to find counteracting US advantages. With little else available, they must look to the aging B-52 bomber fleet.

Arms control experts have made a silk purse out of the "sowish" B-52 by equating one such aircraft equipped with cruise missiles to a heavy ICBM. One B-52 equals one mammoth Soviet SS-18, supposedly.[55] This is a specious comparison. The Soviets have defenses against both B-52s and cruise missiles; the United States has none against the SS-18, which can strike its targets in minutes, while US bombers take hours. B-52s are based near the US coast where they are vulnerable to submarine-launched missiles; however, the SS-18s are in hardened silos deep within the Soviet Union. Even so, the United States would need an additional 460 heavy bombers to equal Soviet throw weight.

- Numbers of Warheads. A simple measure, but very dependent on accurate intelligence, is the total number of warheads on each side. Warhead numbers are a good measure of warfighting potential,[56] since the more warheads, the greater the number of military targets an aggressor can strike. Because of performance uncertainty, two or three warheads must be fired at a target to provide confidence in destroying it. In the mid-1980s each superpower had about 10,000 warheads. Although this is ignored by many strategic analysts, I note the growing number of third nation warheads. Between France, Great Britain and China, these nations might hold 2000-4000 missile warheads in the 1990s.[57]

To be sure, warhead numbers are meaningful only in the context of their targets.[58] But just because the Soviet Union assigns a company of troops to guard a vodka plant doesn't make it a meaningful target. Significant military target lists are far more restricted. Four basic classes of targets stand out:

1. Military and civilian leadership
2. Strategic offensive forces (SOF)
3. Other critical military targets such as naval bases (OMT or CMT)
4. War-supporting industries. There are many different lists of these targets.[59] Targets are best represented by "aim-points." Most targets are single aimpoints, but some, such as large military bases, might entail several.

These values suggest that both sides have enough warheads to strike most, if not all, of the opponent's military forces. Figure 6 on p. 75, showing strategic warhead numbers for both super-powers, suggests that each has stopped adding warheads. To me this indicates the individual goal was warfighting. The numbers of warheads on each side is sufficient, even optimum, for this mili-tary mission.

- Strategic Nuclear Delivery Vehicles (SNDVs). Known by the acronym "snydvees" to insiders, SNDVs have been a central parameter in 1980s arms talks. As individual weapons carriers, bomber or missile, came to carry greater numbers of warheads, their importance as a separate meas-ure also grew. SNDVs are important in first-strike and second-strike calculations. Each SNDV is a first-strike tar-get. Both superpowers had about 2500 in the 1980s:

Table 3. Strategic Nuclear Delivery Vehicles

	US	USSR
Targetable SNDVs (ICBMs, bombers)	1,500	2,000
Untargetable SNDVs (Alert bombers, sea- and mobile missiles)	1,000	500
MIRV ratio, warheads per SNDV	4	5
Defense Effectiveness*	0	.2

*Based on Soviet SA-12s, air defenses, and ABMs. The United States is, effectively, undefended.

- Hard-Target Kill Capability. If SNDVs represent first-strike targets, this measure is relevant to a side's ability to hit them. To compute this measure one adds the number of *missile* warheads with sufficient accuracy to crack enemy missile silos. (Bombers are ignored; they're easy.) The Soviet Union has a big advantage, 6000 hard-target killers versus 1500 US Minuteman III warheads. In the mid-1980s the Minuteman III warheads were our only hard-target killers. With 1500 warheads, the United States couldn't effectively target the 2500 Soviet SNDVs, most of which are in hardened targets. In the 1990s the United States will have numerous MX and sub-launched D-5 warheads with hard-target kill capability. It remains to be seen whether it will have sufficient numbers of these weapons for even a theoretical first-strike capability.

- Equivalent Weapons. Many people have tried to come up with a composite index to measure total warfighting potential.[60] An equivalent weapons measure would include the number and yield of warheads, their accuracy, and the characteristics of their targets. It is hard to derive such a number. Without knowing each side's war aims, it's impossible to quantify their overall warfighting potential.

Static indices have two weaknesses. First, they ignore the human dimension. Wars, even nuclear ones, are not fought by computers. People, with all their shortcomings, fight other people. They lack data and have emotions. The fact that his family lives a half kilometer from a SNDV will surely affect the nuclear warrior. Second, comparisons of numbers ignore what Clausewitz called "friction" or the "fog of war."[61] Nothing in war ever works out as it was planned. Even without "nuclear winter," nuclear conflict will not lack in "fog" or "friction."

War Gaming and Simulation

We can never know how people would actually act in crises prior to nuclear war—let alone during that war. We can, however, examine human behavior related to some specific aspect of nuclear war. The only tool for this is the war game, the second form of strategic analysis.

Many groups conduct those, and some of the best are the war games conducted by the Joint Chiefs of Staff (JCS). JCS war games often involve those who would actually make the critical decisions in a crisis.[62] They try to place participants under the pressure of dealing with actual enemies. Typically two teams assemble—a "blue" and a "red" team, with each having about ten players. Players may adopt roles, or actually hold the positions as Chairman of the Joint Chiefs of Staff, Secretary of Defense, President, or others. A control team manages play, and presents the sides with a crisis—for example, a Mideast war. The sides must decide what to do within a fixed time limit. Games may take days, and follow-on analysis months. Out of the game results valuable information flows about human behavior in crises, what "wins" and what doesn't, and perhaps some information on how to avoid actions that might lead to nuclear war.

Every effort is made to simulate a real crisis. The JCS gameroom is in the sub-basement of the Pentagon, where participants are held incommunicado during the game. But no game can "fool" the participants' emotions. Only real crises can place the knowledge in players' minds that the fate of the nation rests on their actions in the next few minutes.

Practical Estimates

The third form of strategic analysis is the practical estimate. Sophisticated mathematics can illuminate, darkly, the world situation after a nuclear exchange. Mathematical uncertainty can crudely model the fog of war. A "Red Integrated Strategic Operations Plan—RISOP" can represent the best US estimates of Soviet war aims. It can be played against the US "Strategic Integrated Operations Plan—SIOP." These plans include some notion of war aims, and victory. I examine possible Soviet war aims in chapter 4. Here I review possible US war aims.

As I described earlier, US objectives are to deter war by presenting the Soviet Union with defeat. This means a postwar world where their military objectives have failed and their relative strength, compared to the enemy, is unfavorable. Basic US war aims fall into four categories:[63]

1. Limit damage to the United States and its allies.

2. Defeat Soviet war aims.

3. Terminate hostilities on terms favorable to the United States.

4. Seek a decisive solution to a protracted conflict. For example, the United States might use nuclear weapons to defeat a Soviet attack on Western Europe.

Specific strategies to accomplish these war aims are numerous and controversial. Regardless of strategy, the United States measures success using a parameter called Damage Expectancy or DE.[64] Strategic planners measure it against a specific target set. It is the percentage of a target set the United States could destroy *after* absorbing a Soviet first strike. For example, there are about 500 Soviet airfields. If the United States destroyed 200 of these following a Soviet first strike, our DE would be 0.40.

Most US targeting strategies take one of four forms. Each focuses on a different facet of Soviet power or Soviet war aims.

1. *Destruction of Soviet Long-Range Nuclear Forces.* Some Soviet nuclear might would have gone into a first strike, but the Soviet Union would also maintain a reserve force. US strategists, steeped in MAD theory, have tended to identify this reserve as an "assured destruction" force, and many have worried that it could hold the US population hostage to deter any response to the initial Soviet strike.[65] A Soviet strike directed solely against the US military, particularly if confined to nuclear retaliatory forces, would kill millions—20 million by competent estimates.[66] This would be an unprecedented blow to the United States, and the fate of the remaining 200 million people, vulnerable to a Soviet countervalue response, would certainly weigh heavily on the President's mind. He might prefer capitulation to countering the initial Soviet attack.

One way to limit this blackmail threat would be to destroy it in our retaliation. This was part of the US "damage limiting" concept of the 1960s.[67] But in the 1980s the Soviet Union had enough nuclear power for immense reserves. Moreover, these reserves are mobile and defended. I conclude that offensive damage limiting is not a credible option for the 1990s and beyond for our offensive systems. Damage limitation through *defensive* capabilities may be a possibility.

2. *Destroy and Disrupt Soviet Controls.* Few dispute whether the Soviet Union is a centrally controlled state. It is. It also relies on a far more centrally controlled military than the West. These facts present an opportunity. If the United States could destroy the Soviet military command, control and communications (C^3) system, its military leaders might well lose control of the armed forces. The theory goes that, if "decapitated," the Soviet armed forces would last about as long as Marie Antoinette did following her fate on the guillotine. A second, similar possibility has interested many strategists, for example, Colin Gray.[68] Several thousand senior communist party officials—the "Nomenklatura"—run the Soviet Union. Many observers regard, with some justification, the Soviet Union as an occupied empire. As such, it could fragment with the leadership gone. A possible strategy might thus be to target only the Nomenklatura, since Soviet leaders might be more cautious about risking nuclear war if they knew they would be the first to suffer.

Targeting the Nomenklatura might not work, though. Foremost among the problems is the Soviet passive defense system. By conservative estimate the Soviets have hundreds, if not thousands, of deep underground "Fuhrer-bunkers."[69] The United States has only two, the Cheyenne Mountain defense complex in Colorado, and a Presidential emergency command center in the Eastern United States. At the first sign of trouble the Nomenklatura would no doubt retreat into their bunkers.[70] The uncertainty as to how many there are of those is ample evidence of these problems, while another problem is casualties. When not in their bunkers, the Nomenklatura stay in cities, where leaders usually are. There's no way to remove the Nomenklatura without killing tens of millions of people. The casualties would approach McNamara's assured destruction goal of 25 percent of the Soviet population. Such devastation runs counter to US policy. In 1985, US National Security Advisor, William P. Clark, said:

For moral, political and military reasons, the United States does not target the Soviet civilian populations as such. There is no deliberately opaque meaning conveyed by the last two words. We do not threaten the existence of Soviet civilization by threatening Soviet cities. Rather we hold at risk the war making capacity of the Soviet Union—its armed forces, and the industrial capacity to wage war.[71]

More significantly, such devastation defies logic. Neither Soviet military forces nor occupied peoples will be favorably disposed to a revolt favoring the West when it has just finished annihilating millions, along with the senior communist party officials. Many experts believe it was Hitler's brutal policy against the Ukrainian and Russian people which saved Stalin from internal revolt in World War II.[72] Just as German bullets garnered support for the Soviet leadership—so too would US nuclear bombs.

3. *Destroy or Disrupt War-Supporting Industry.* It might be possible to so damage the Soviet economy that it could not recover in any reasonable time. A deliberate strategy to do this gained adherents in the 1970s. Soviet writings have shown some concern with post-nuclear war correlation of economic forces. If Soviet military and economic recovery following a war were slow in comparison with the enemy, that possibility could help deter war. A variant on general economic targeting is to concentrate on war-supporting industry, especially since Soviet writings emphasize the likelihood of a protracted general war. The early likely loss of war-supporting capacity could also help deter war. Some senior US officials pushed an industrial-oriented strategy in the 1970s. General George Brown, Chairman of the Joint Chiefs of Staff, said in 1977, "We do not target population per se any longer. What we are doing now is targeting a war recovery capability."[73]

Economic targeting is as difficult as leadership targeting. The Soviet Union protects its industry through increasingly effective civil defenses. Targeting industry is like targeting cities—it is done because that is where the factories are. Finally, it is a questionable assumption that Soviet industry would be more damaged than Western industry. World War II showed that the Soviet Union can recover rapidly after losing much of its industrial capacity.

4. *Destroy or Degrade Other Military Forces.* The basis of Soviet power is, and always has been, integrated military might. Ultimately, the Red Army must win the war. A good Western strategy would be to destroy or weaken it so that it would lose in battle. This is a sensible goal—but can we do it?

A simple model shows that the West lacks the offensive forces to effectively attack Soviet military might. A key reason for this is Soviet defenses—passive as well as active. Soviet air defenses are massive—they spend as much on them as they do on offensive forces. Passive defenses, "Fuhrer-bunkers," pro-·tect their military leadership and command systems. Missile defenses in the form of the Moscow ABM and SA-12 anti-tactical missile system provide increasing defense protection against Western missiles.[74]

For my example calculation I'll restrict myself to missile forces. Bombers, cruise missiles (and defenses against these) can be treated in a similar manner. For simplicity, I equate a cruise-missile-armed bomber to an ICBM and assign some effectiveness to Soviet air defenses, while US defenses can be ignored. The calculation starts with a list of static parameters:

	US	USSR
1. Strategic Offensive Missiles—SNDVs (fixed land-based—assumed targetable)	X	X'
2. Untargetable missiles—SNDVs (sea-based and mobile land-based)	XX	XX'
3. Warheads per offensive missile (multiple warheads per missile—MIRVs)	Y	Y'
4. Defense effectiveness (0%=0, 100%=1)	A	A'

From these parameters I can calculate how many US targets would be destroyed in a first strike. I assume that the Soviet Union would strike both at targetable offensive missiles and other military targets such as air bases, submarine pens, and troop concentrations—anything which would put them in a better military situation after the strike. I also assume a conservative Soviet targeting plan—they would fire three warheads at each target to ensure success. The total number of targets the Soviets would destroy is represented by "P", where:

$$P = (X' + XX') \times Y' \times (1-A) / 3 .$$

The Soviet war planner is interested in how many non-missile targets he has destroyed. He separates this from missile targets in order to compute the damage done to US non-retaliatory war-fighting capability. This number is simply:

$$P_{US} = P - X .$$

This ends the first strike. Now I will calculate how many Soviet military targets the United States hits in its retaliation. To make it simple, I assume that the Soviet Union used all of its fixed missiles in the first strike. Since these missiles would be vulnerable to a retaliatory strike, it's likely that the Soviets would see the wisdom in a "use them or lose them" policy. Of course, this also means that the United States doesn't need to target Soviet fixed missiles in its retaliation—but can focus on other Soviet military targets.

Because the United States could lose much of its force in the first strike, and because its missiles have better reliability and accuracy, I assume that the United States would only aim two warheads at each Soviet target. The number of Soviet targets destroyed in the US retaliation is given by the number "Q."

Thus

$$Q = (X - (X' + XX) \times Y' \times (1 - A) + XX) \times Y \times (1 - A') / 2 .$$

This looks complicated, but two things make it simple. The Soviet Union has so many hard-target killers that none of the US land-based missiles would survive, so the first part of the equation can be ignored. Moreover, the United States has no defense, so the second part goes away too. The final number of Soviet military facilities destroyed in the retaliation is simply:

$$Q_{USSR} = XX \times Y \times (1 - A') / 2 .$$

This is the number of targets we hit with our mobile land-based and sea-based missile warheads reduced by the effectiveness of Soviet defenses.

If the United States hopes to deter the Soviet Union, we should end up better off militarily than they. Or, put mathematically:

$$Q_{USSR} > P_{US}.$$

Can we meet this criterion? Emphatically no! To show why not, I do the following calculation using some approximate numbers characteristic of the mid-1980s.[75]

The results are:

$$P_{US} = 2500, Q_{USSR} = 1600 \ .$$

In their strike the Soviet Union would have effectively wiped out all US military forces, both SNDVs and other military targets. The US retaliation would damage Soviet armed might, but leave about half of it intact. Few would argue that the Soviet Union would have ''won'' the war in a military sense—but they would be in a much stronger military position than their Western adversaries.

These imbalances are not so overwhelming that the United States must fear a Soviet bolt from the blue. Soviet victory in this simple calculation depends on a number of factors. Key among them would be the effectiveness of Soviet defenses. With the Clausewitzian concept of uncertainty in mind—the ''fog of war''— no war, as I noted earlier, could easily prevent the Soviet Union from gaining anything as clear-cut as my calculation suggests. However, in-depth calculations taking many factors into account, including uncertainty, show that current US Damage Expectancy (DE) against a wide range of targets is about 0.6—in line with my simple calculation. A DE of 0.9 is required for anything like an effective military warfighting strategy.[76] To achieve this DE goal, the United States must increase significantly its offensive forces *or* add effective defenses. Neither is likely in the political climate of the 1990s.

The most serious problem with these analyses is the fog of war itself. I ask readers to place themselves in the shoes of the Soviet General Secretary or the US President. Neither leader is likely to have had experience in strategic analysis, and one, or both, might be too uncertain to react quickly and decisively in a crisis. Faced with incomprehension at a moment of swift-moving perceived disaster, they might react by asking their military leaders to retaliate immediately with all the force at their command. Out of such circumstances, I fear, World War III could emerge, despite thousands of pages of careful strategic analysis. None of the approaches I've outlined—not static comparisons, not war games, and not sophisticated exchange calculations—can address this issue adequately.

The Best Defense Is a Good Offense

From the preceding analysis it should be clear that defenses can play an important role. They can defend retaliatory forces or other military targets. Many of the United States' strategic analysts believe that defending retaliatory forces is the best defensive mission. Former Defense Secretary Harold Brown believes it is the only reasonable possibility.[77] Robert McNamara calls defending ICBMs "Star Wars II" and identifies this as the real goal of the SDI. He is appalled by the very thought of defending people, which he identifies as "Star Wars I," a perfect defense believed feasible by only President Reagan.[78] In an interview with McNamara I raised the possibility of the defense-reliant deterrent I discuss in the next chapter. McNamara rejected this possibility with a colorful metaphor.[79]

There is little debate whether defenses can defend a retaliatory force. They can. The issue is whether such defense is the best way to protect retaliatory forces. But, more important, is it "stabilizing"? Skeptics of defenses, like Harold Brown, often cite ways other than defenses to enhance offensive system survivability—mobile ICBMs, more submarine-launched missiles, stealth cruise missiles, and others. Clausewitzian views of defenses give rise to the instability argument. The Prussian General clearly identified defense as a superior form of war.[80] He was not referring to a pure defense, which he said, "would be completely contrary to the idea of war, since it would mean that only one side was waging it."[81] Clausewitz viewed defense as the key part of offensive operations—either as a means of buying time to gather offensive strength or to protect oneself from enemy counteroffensives.[82] Defense as a subordinate part of offensive operations is very much in the minds of those who reject the SDI.

Robert McNamara outlines the offensive character of defenses in his book *Blundering into Disaster*, the title accurately representing his unbiased and unemotional view of the SDI.

> Why will the Soviets suspect that Star Wars II (defense of missile silos) is designed to support a first-strike strategy? Because a leaky umbrella offers no protection in a downpour but is quite useful in a drizzle. That is, such a defense

would collapse under a full scale Soviet first strike but
might cope adequately with the depleted Soviet Forces
which had survived a US first strike.[83]

The Soviet Union has obviously read Clausewitz, if not the
views of SDI critics. In one of their anti-SDI publications, *Star
Wars, Delusion and Dangers*, the Soviets make the statement:
"In this set-up ('Star Wars'), the purpose of the space shield is
to frustrate the Soviet Union's retaliatory strike, to 'finish off' at
launch those of its missiles that survive the nuclear first strike of
the United States of America."[84]

Of course, these arguments have little bearing in reality. The
United States does not have a first-strike capability, and is unlikely
to get one for political reasons. More important, my analysis made
it clear that with roughly *equal* defenses on both sides, defense
helps the defender almost much as the attacker. There is little danger of unilateral US defenses—the converse is much more likely.
The Soviet Union already has significant strategic defense.[85]

Is there a way to illustrate the potential instability? Lieutenant
General Glenn Kent developed an approach which I will call the
"Kent" diagram.[86] As illustrated in Figure 7, I plot both sides'
defensive capabilities. If these defenses get good enough, we have
"assured survival" for the population. A similar analysis is possible from a retaliation-based deterrent perspective. If those defenses
are effective, militarily insignificant damage would occur—a military form of "assured survival." At intermediate defense levels, a
side could still avoid significant damage by striking first at the
opponent's retaliatory forces. A "conditional survival" situation
results. One side has sufficient defenses so that it can survive by
striking first and using the remaining defenses to mop up the
"ragged" retaliation. This provides a temptation for a first strike.
It is stable, but terrible for the disadvantaged party. A more unstable situation exists when both sides have enough defenses for conditional survival—in the Kent diagram their conditional survival
curves overlap. Either side could win by striking first, but must
fear a similar act by the other. In this case the *pressure* for a first
strike is great and the deterrent most unstable.

One of the criticisms of moving to a defense-reliant deterrent is that it cannot be reached without passing through this
most unstable region.[87]

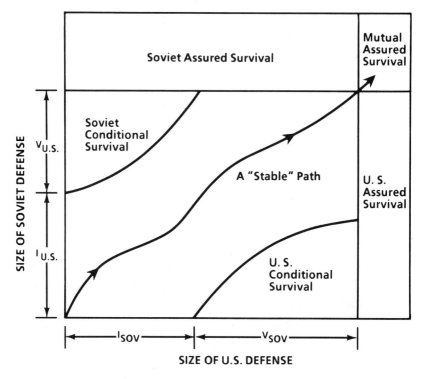

Source: C. Max, P. Banks, et al. *Deployment Stability of Strategic Forces* (McLean, VA: JASON/MITRE, October 1986)

Figure 7. The "Glenn Kent" Stability Diagram. Named after retired Lt. Gen. Glenn Kent, the diagram plots, as a function of US and Soviet defense effectiveness, the type of deterrent operating in each region. Offenses are held fixed on both sides while defenses vary. I is the number of invulnerable (not targetable by the opponent) RVs on both sides; V is the number of vulnerable ones. The conditional survival zones are regions where each side will suffer no retaliatory damage if it strikes first, but would suffer damage if it were to strike second. A "stable" force configuration is defined as one in which conditional regions of the two sides do not touch or overlap.

One of the curious aspects of debate over the wisdom of US strategic defenses is critics' attention to the instability outlined above. Yet, there is seldom much concern from these critics over Soviet defenses. Those defenses are formidable and growing in the 1990s. At a level I estimate to be at least 20 percent effective now, we may already be entering a regime of Soviet conditional survival—at least from a military perspective. The West should take note of this development and be less concerned with US-induced potential instability and more with Soviet-caused reality.

The Bottom Line

US deterrent strategy must be based on a plausible victory concept. If the reader prefers a less emotional characterization, this might be Soviet defeat. However, the United States and its allies must face these facts:

1. The West does not have the forces to present the Soviet Union with *any* plausible prospect of Western victory.

2. The West is unlikely to recover a military-based deterrent due to political constraints. The people will not support building the necessary nuclear forces.

3. The addition of defenses to Western nuclear-offensive strategies could help redress the balance. Conversely, the inevitable Soviet defenses can negate any advantage Western defenses might win.

4. Nuclear offensive forces cannot be the key to Western security in the decades ahead.

5. We must consider an alternative, non-nuclear deterrent strategy.

3. NON-NUCLEAR DETERRENCE

Consider a 2400-year-old strategy.

For to win one hundred victories in one hundred battles is not the acme of skill. To subdue the enemy without fighting is the acme of skill.

Thus, what is of supreme importance in war is to attack the enemy's strategy.

Next best is to disrupt his alliances.

The next best is to attack his army.

The worst policy is to attack cities. Attack cities only when there is no alternative.[1]

> Sun Tzu
> circa 400 B.C.

Contrast the ancient Chinese ideas with a 150-year-old approach.

If for the moment we consider the pure concept of war, we should have to say that the political purpose of war had no connection with war itself; for if war is an act of violence meant to force the enemy to do our will its aim would have *always* and *solely* to be to overcome the enemy and disarm him.

We should at once distinguish between three things, three broad objectives, which between them cover everything: the armed forces, the country, and the enemy's will.... Since of the three objectives named, it is the fighting forces that assure the safety of the country, the natural sequence would be to destroy them first, and then subdue the country. Having achieved these two goals and exploiting their own position of strength, we can bring the enemy to the peace table.[2]

> Karl von Clausewitz
> 1818

We should also review an upstart 40-year-old strategy:

Thus far the chief purpose of our military establishment has been to win wars. From now on its chief purpose must be to avert them. It can have almost no other useful purpose.[3]

Bernard Brodie
1946

When President Reagan asked the American people the following question on March 23, 1983, he chose the 2400-year-old approach: "What if free people could live secure in the knowledge that their security did not rest on the threat of instant US retaliation to deter a Soviet attack, that we could intercept and destroy strategic missiles before they reached our soil and that of our Allies?"[4]

Denying Enemy Plans

Strategies relying on defenses have surfaced several times since 1945. Each time they triggered vigorous emotional debates. Each time the defensive strategy lost. Sun Tzu's words reveal the reason. His strategy places the two non-defensive approaches to nuclear warfare most popular in the United States at the bottom of the list. Clausewitz advocated a warfighting strategy directed against the enemy armed might. Sun Tzu thought this was almost the worst thing one could do. MAD, of course, assumes war will never happen. But if it does, we would do the worst possible thing on Sun Tzu's list—attack enemy cities. It is no wonder that critics of strategic defense react so strongly, since defensive strategy urges the exact opposite of their approaches.

Why should the United States consider a new strategy? After all, we have not had a major war since World War II, the West is prosperous and there is no imminent threat to our security. Deterrence seems to have worked. Why question success? A good question indeed! But there is also a good answer. MAD places war prevention above all else. War has been the ultimate remedy to evil in the past. Without recourse to war there is no way to redress the misdeeds of our potential adversaries. Worse yet, MAD is silent on what to do if deterrence fails—as I believe it could. Throughout history nations have tried to deter war. In the past decades many acted as if deterrence would last forever. Some have sought answers in history—what, for example, deterred war in centuries past: a strong military, the threat of state-sponsored murder, stout walls, diplomacy? The results of these studies are sobering.[5] Nothing seems to deter war for long—not armies, not threats of death, not even strong walls or wide oceans. MAD's answer— the end of the world—cannot be our answer.

Nuclear warriors have an answer—be ready to fight and win a nuclear war. A war-winning capability can then be used to frighten would-be aggressors and transgressors. Perhaps we could fight and win a nuclear war. But I fear that both politics and technology preclude this approach to deterrence. The warriors offer little solace to us if deterrence fails. Our great-grandchildren might be thankful that the United States fought and won World War III. But I doubt that that war's participants would share those views. However, a defensive strategy offers a third way.

Defense-reliant deterrence's first goal is to discover the potential enemy's strategic plans. Our defensive capabilities must then demonstrate convincingly that those plans will fail and that the aggressor's goals will be unmet.

Long ago the Chinese General Sun Tzu wrote about how to attack enemy strategies: "It is a doctrine of war not to assume the enemy will not come, but rather to rely on one's readiness to meet him; not to presume that he will not attack, but rather to make one's self invincible."[6] To this end Sun Tzu gave the key, "invincibility lies in the defense."[7]

I maintain that Soviet strategy is based on three elements: disruption of Western cohesiveness and will; strategic offensive forces to destroy Western warfighting ability; and the Red Army's capability to take and control territory. Strategic defenses only address the middle one of these—Soviet offensive forces. This chapter shows how to neutralize those. But we should not ignore other Soviet strategic elements. In several places throughout this book I have stated that advanced space technologies can counter the Red Army. But the details on how to do this, as well as how we might counter the even more formidable Soviet political attack, are beyond this book's scope.

In an interview with former Secretary of Defense Robert McNamara, he challenged me to produce a coherent set of criteria for defense-reliant deterrence.[8] This chapter is designed to answer that challenge. To summarize my approach, US aims should be as follows.

1. Discover the strategic war aims of Soviet offensive forces and deploy or demonstrate defensive capability sufficient to defeat those aims should war occur.

2. Develop technical capabilities which can defeat the war aims of any strategy which relies on weapons of mass destruction.

3. Deploy sufficient defenses to ensure that the United States and its allies can survive as functioning societies against enemy mass destruction attacks.

4. Ensure that a transition from strategies relying on weapons of mass destruction can be made without an increased war threat to the people of the United States.

Defenses in the Nuclear Age

Nuclear weapons had scarcely been invented when the search for defensive counters began. Since the end of the Second World War, strategic defense adherents have repeatedly proposed large defense investments. They have achieved little success in their efforts. On the one hand, they must contend with the prevailing US belief in the supremacy of offensive nuclear weapons. Under this mindset defenses take a back seat—serving solely to defend offensive forces. When resources are tight, as they inevitably are, we forgo them. On the other hand, defense advocates are confronted with a US intellectual community that regards their views as heresy.

The strategic defense debate began in 1945. General H. H. "Hap" Arnold, Chief of Army Air Forces during World War II, gave a revealing viewpoint on defenses against atomic bombs in his final war report. Foreseeing ICBMs, he stated: "Although there now appear to be insurmountable difficulties in an active defense against future atomic projectiles similar to the German V-2 but armed with atomic explosives, this condition should only intensify our efforts to find an effective means of defense.''[9]

But a few sentences later General Arnold left no doubt where he thought our priorities should lie: "While this country must employ all of its physical and moral force in the cause of peace, it must recognize that real security against atomic weapons in the visible future will rest on our ability to take immediate offensive action with overwhelming force."[10]

In the late 1940s some military officers tried to press for intensive defensive efforts and political leaders were optimistic that effective defenses could be built.[11] But academics, such as Bernard Brodie and many physicists, were almost uniformly hostile to them. Brodie's view on defense usefulness is summed up in his pithy 1946 statement: "No adequate answer has yet been found for the bullet."[12] Many factors—focus on offensive forces, tight budgets, academic animosity, and the lack of a credible Soviet nuclear threat—crushed any strong US interest in strategic defense for almost a decade after the war.

The Soviet atomic bomb explosion in 1949 and hydrogen bomb test in 1953 changed everything. I do not intend to provide an exhaustive history of US strategic defense work. Instead, I will give a broad-brush review of the oft-contentious debate over strategic defenses. The public arguments tended to focus on technical details of specific defensive systems. But the root of the debate was always philosophical.

An outstanding, and unfortunately unpublished, summary of strategic defense debates of the 1950s and 1960s appears in a 1969 Ph.D. dissertation by Edward Jayne.[13] For an update to the 1980s, I recommend an article by David Swartz.[14] There were four major cycles in these debates, pitting advocates of the three schools of deterrence against one another. These debates must be distinguished from the cycles I discussed in Chapter 1. The MAD versus warfighting discussions played out largely within the defense intellectual community. The arguments I discuss here were public, emotional, and divisive.

Interservice Rivalry (1957-1960)

The Army and the Air Force developed air defense systems in the early 1950s to stop Soviet bombers. The Air Force fielded its BOMARC air defense missile and the Army its Nike series. The 1953 Soviet hydrogen bomb explosion, signaling true superpower status for that nation, also triggered a US Air Force-Army fight. As early as 1950, groups of scientists at MIT had proposed a defense-reliant US strategy as opposed to an offensive approach.[15] By 1953 a number of scientific and consultant groups were advocating strong, if not dominant, US defense reliance. The Army was an enthusiastic cheerleader for these efforts. The Air Force made its negative opinion clear in blunt statements, for example the 1953 Congressional testimony by Air Force Under Secretary James H. Douglas:

> As to the question "should we place reliance on air defense as our best protection" my answer is that we should not ... Science gives it (defense) great possibilities. But let us avoid the dangers of thinking of it as our best protection ... To do so would be to put second things first and divert us from concentrating our attention on the long-range atomic striking power.[16]

By 1955 both the Army and the Air Force had begun missile defense programs. The Army approach, called Nike Zeus, was to upgrade its Nike Hercules anti-aircraft system. The Air Force Wizard program, on the other hand, was a new approach. The interservice battle was on. Wizard emphasized long-range, 1000-mile intercept, while Nike Zeus was a shorter range concept. The Army won a minor victory on 26 November 1956. Secretary of Defense Wilson split the program—the Army got the point defense mission, the Air Force got the tougher area defense job. By late 1957 the Army was ready for full-scale development and deployment of Nike Zeus. The Air Force, losing and not terribly enthusiastic about defense anyway, fought back.

The Air Force used two basic arguments. In support of its offense-oriented strategy, the Air Force identified defense of Strategic Air Command bases as the only useful defense mission. Even this wasn't needed, they said, since there were cheaper ways to ensure bomber survivability, such as dispersal under warning.[17] The Air Force also enlisted technical arguments against Nike Zeus. Since the Zeus intercepted warheads outside the atmosphere, it could be fooled by lightweight decoys in space which looked just like warheads.[18] Although the Army managed to get the Air Force Wizard project canceled in 1958, relegating the Air Force to improving radar capabilities, the latter service had denigrated Nike Zeus enough to ensure non-deployment.[19] During the remainder of the Eisenhower administration the Army failed to deploy Zeus—despite a 1958 end run using sympathetic members of Congress.[20]

To stop Nike Zeus the Air Force enlisted some strange bedfellows—the scientists. In his 1959 State of the Union message, President Eisenhower placed all ABM research under a civilian agency—the Advanced Research Projects Agency, or ARPA.[21] ARPA scientists and their White House colleagues helped the Air Force devise marvelous countermeasures to Nike Zeus.[22] The Air Force would soon come to rue the day it sold its soul to the scientists.

Making the Argument Public (1965-1969)

Defensive strategy advocates hoped for victory when the Kennedy administration adopted flexible response as official US policy. As I discussed in chapter 2, the Army played a key role in pushing that strategy. It certainly appeared that Defense Secretary Robert McNamara's twin goals, assured destruction and damage limitation, required some defensive capabilities. The Army thought that Nike Zeus was ideal for limiting damage and pushed for a deployment. The Air Force, beginning to worry about ICBM survivability, became more receptive to ABM deployments as a way of protecting their assured destruction forces.[23]

Why, then, did the United States not deploy strategic missile defenses in the early 1960s? The scientific community proved to be the joker in the deck. Scientists within the administration had lots of technical excuses for deferring deployment. A key victory was assured when the scientists persuaded McNamara that an ABM should not be deployed unless it could defeat not only current missiles but future developments as well. This unfortunate albatross hung around the necks of strategic defenders well into the 1980s. Surprisingly, US offensive deployments never seem to be judged against possible future Soviet defenses! Two arguments against Nike Zeus popped up time and again.[24] First, the mechanically steered radars could be overloaded by a large attack—unable to track more than a few objects simultaneously. Second, sophisticated Soviet decoys, available at some unspecified future date, were said to be able to fool and exhaust Nike Zeus. The scientists insisted that more research was needed to solve these problems. Internal DOD scientists killed Zeus with an oft-used trick. "Let's do more Research and Development," which might be translated into "Research forever, Deploy never!"

Arms control, the darling of the Kennedy administration, was a potent weapon against ABM. Defense-minded senators tried to use the ABM research program as a reason to reject the 1963 atmospheric nuclear test ban treaty.[25] This clumsy attempt further convinced the scientific community, always fond of "dialogue" with the Soviets, that ABM was the enemy of arms control. The Federation of American Scientists, spearheaded by Nobel Laureate and Manhattan Project alumnus Hans Bethe, led the assault. They convinced McNamara that ABMs would upset the delicate strategic balance which they viewed to be MAD-based.

A final nail in the Nike Zeus's coffin came from McNamara's systems analysts. The Glenn Kent analyses of 1964[26] cited in chapters 1 and 2 showed that ABMs were not the most cost-effective way to limit damage. The studies concluded that ABMs must be part of an overall damage-limiting package—including anti-submarine warfare, air defense, counterforce targeting, and civil defense. Civil defense invariably turned out tops in cost effectiveness. Thus, missile defense was held hostage to a large-scale civil defense. The political unacceptability of civil defense thus blocked any moves toward active missile defense.

By the late 1960s, two new factors entered the strategic scene. Soviet strategic missile defenses became undeniable, and they were growing. On the US side research and development had solved many of the technical objections of the early 1960s.

Soviet interest in air defense and civil defense has always been high, as I will discuss in Chapter 4. The Soviet Union probably began anti-missile work about the time they started on long-range missiles. In the early 1960s, their work began to pay off. On 6 September 1961 the Soviet Union live-fired and successfully intercepted a ballistic missile warhead.[27] The reader mustn't miss the significance of the term "live fire." This was the actual interception of a live nuclear warhead with a nuclear-armed interceptor detonating to destroy it. The 1961 Soviet test series contained several of these experiments—an uniquely valuable set of data to this day.[28] By October, 1962 the Soviet Union was confident enough of nationwide defense possibilities for Soviet Defense Minister Malinovskiy to tell the 23rd Congress of the Communist Party of the Soviet Union that Russian ABMs were ready for American ICBMs. By 1965 Marshal Malinovskiy would brag that, "The complex and extremely important problem of destroying any enemy rockets in flight has been solved."[29]

American discussion centered on three possible Soviet ABM systems. In 1961 the Leningrad air defense system (the "Griffon" system) appeared to some US analysts to have ABM potential.[30] Nike Zeus advocates in the Senate tried, unsuccessfully, to use the Soviet system as a reason for near-term US deployments.[31] However, general expert opinion was that the Leningrad Griffon system was at best capable only against short- and medium-range ballistic missiles.[32] The second Soviet system was unmistakably an ABM. The Soviets paraded their long-range Galosh interceptor through Moscow in November 1964.[33] By 1965 they had begun to construct the Moscow Galosh ABM system. A third Soviet effort is still a mystery, but potentially had the largest strategic importance. Whereas the Moscow and Leningrad defenses were basically "point" defenses of those cities, the third system appeared to be an area defense. In the mid 1960s the Soviets began deploying a swath of radars and interceptors across the US ICBM attack corridor. This system, code named Tallinn because it first appeared near the Estonian capital city of that name, may or may not have had ballistic missile defense capabilities.[34] It used an upgraded anti-aircraft defense missile—the SA-5. If Tallinn was an area missile defense, it could protect much of the European USSR.

By 1967 Secretary McNamara was confronted with unmistakable evidence of a massive Soviet ABM commitment. US engineers had also solved the two main technical shortcomings of Nike Zeus. In the early 1960s the Air Force developed phased array radars which could replace the old steerable dish radars. With no moving parts, they could be pointed at targets electronically rather than mechanically. They could thus simultaneously track hundreds of targets. The second problem, warhead decoys, also had a 1960s solution. If an interceptor missile was fast enough, it might delay launch until after the attacking warheads and decoys reentered the atmosphere. It is possible to distinguish real warheads from decoys. Decoys weigh a small fraction of a warhead's weight and they slow down much faster due to air friction once they get into the atmosphere. This effect gives away the real warheads, which can then be attacked by the interceptor. In 1963 the United States began development of just such an "inside the atmosphere" or endo-atmospheric interceptor—the Nike-X. By 1967 the Nike-X, or Sprint, was ready to go.

Soviet defenses and advancing technology convinced strategic defense advocates in Congress and the Joint Chiefs of Staff that it was time to move ahead. There was a critical meeting in Austin, Texas on 6 December 1966 during which JCS Chairman Wheeler convinced President Johnson to approve deployment of an ABM. Secretary McNamara strongly opposed this move.[35]

Out of McNamara's defeat at the hands of defense professionals grew the seeds of his later victory. During the December 1966 meeting he had extracted President Johnson's commitment to a vigorous arms control initiative to accompany the ABM deployment. Indeed, ABM deployment was not to proceed unless arms control failed. McNamara used his ace in the hole (the scientists) in January 1967, bringing prior DOD research directors and White House science advisors to the President to argue against ABM deployments directed at the Soviet Union.

McNamara's initial arms control overtures failed. On 23 June 1967 Soviet Prime Minister Kosygin met with President Johnson and McNamara at the Glassboro summit. The Soviet leader definitively rejected arms control of defenses. According to McNamara, Kosygin forcefully pointed out that, "Defense is moral; offense is immoral!"[36] According to other reports Kosygin called McNamara an "immoral capitalist."[37] Arms control, at least for a time, looked discouraging. President Johnson ordered McNamara to proceed with ABM deployment.

The reluctant Defense Secretary sought far and wide for the minimum ABM which would mollify the defense community. The June 1967 Chinese entry into the nuclear club provided just the ticket—an anti-Chinese ABM. The system proposed by McNamara, called Sentinel, was to provide a light area defense against Chinese attack. Sentinel was actually two systems, the short-range Sprint interceptor and associated radars, and a long-range "outside the atmosphere" or exo-atmospheric interceptor, the Spartan. Spartan was an upgraded version of the old Nike Zeus.

McNamara did not favor any ABM. In his speech announcing the Sentinel deployment decision on 18 September 1967 he stressed the danger of an ABM-induced arms race. The following exerpt from that San Francisco speech seems a strange way to advocate a new system: "Our greatest deterrent ... is not a massive, costly, but highly penetrable ABM shield, but rather a fully credible offensive assured destruction capability."[38]

Although the defense professionals had won within the administration, the battle for ABM was far from over. In late 1968 an election campaign was in full swing and the Vietnam War was an increasingly emotional issue. In this environment ABM deployments became a big political football. On the left stood the scientific community, imbued with MAD theology. It aligned itself with liberal elements of the political spectrum who were seeking to shift funds from military programs to social spending. On the other side was an alliance of defense professionals faced with growing Soviet nuclear power. To these people, ABMs, combined with other initiatives, were a potent military counter to the Soviets. Between January 1968 and August 1969 the debate raged.

In what appears on reflection to be a Machiavellian stroke of genius, McNamara approved the first ABM deployment for Boston. The United States would have had an easier time deploying nuclear weapons around Moscow than deploying them near the very heartland of liberal and scientific assumed superiority. The result was classic—massive "public" protests over ABM in Boston during October 1968. The incoming Nixon administration faced this problem at the start of 1969.

President Nixon's ABM solution became public on 14 March 1969.[39] He changed the system name to "Safeguard" and moved the short-range Sprint sites away from cities. Safeguard resembled Sentinel in most respects except for its mission. The new system's top priority was right out of the retaliation-based deterrent bible—ABMs would protect land-based retaliatory forces from a Soviet first strike. Population defense was only a secondary goal—aimed principally against Chinese ICBMs or accidental enemy launches. President Nixon stressed that Safeguard was not intended, nor should it appear to be intended, as a defense of the American people against a major Soviet strike. The thinking was that a heavy defense of the population might look to an opponent like preparations for a first strike. It's ironic that, like the 1980s, the same logic didn't apply to Soviet air and missile defenses, which were far heavier than any US defenses.

Few voices were raised in the late 1960s in support of defending the American people. But there were some notable exceptions. D. G. Brennan, a physicist, wrote an article in a pro-Safeguard compendium entitled "The Case for Population Defense."[40] Dr. Brennan's arguments reappeared in the 1980s, but they were roundly rejected by even the ABM advocates of the 1960s.

ABM opponents were as united and committed in the 1960s as they are in the 1990s. Led by congressional liberals like Senator Kennedy of Massachusetts and senior scientists, mostly physicists, their arguments were coherent and well publicized[41]—much better presented and better disseminated than the arguments of the ABM advocates. The principal arguments did not change in the 1980s; they were in the 1960s, as they are now, more strategic and theological than technical. Characteristically, the scientists "cashed in" on their scientific credibility, interweaving technical irrelevancies with their political arguments. Their principal arguments were three, as outlined below:

1. There was no sensible mission for ABMs. Four possible ABM missions had been discussed.[42] The critics dismissed each of those:

> **a.** Heavy population defense. This was dismissed as technically impossible. Under MAD logic, the Soviets could

always preserve assured destruction unless the defense was essentially perfect.[43]

b. Light population defense. The scientists dismissed this as technically questionable. They asserted that even third nuclear powers like China could develop effective counter-measures to Safeguard. Besides, the Soviets would have no way of knowing that Safeguard wasn't the first step to a heavy nationwide defense.[44]

c. Defense of the strategic deterrent. This was regarded as feasible, but not needed to protect our assured destruction capacity. The critics pointed out that mobile strategic missiles, both land and sea-based, and launch-on-warning tactics were cheaper ways to ensure our deterrent.[45]

d. Defense against accidental launch. The critics said that this was not worth it. They claimed that the accidental launch of a nuclear-armed defensive missile was a greater danger, and one that could trigger a nuclear war.[46]

2. There would be damage to arms control. ABM critics claimed that the Soviets would respond to a US anti-ballistic missile with an offensive buildup to preserve their assured destruction capacity. Moreover, the Soviets would worry about a US first strike. This environment was asserted to be poor for arms control.[47]

3. There were insurmountable technical problems.

a. By simply building more offensive missiles the Soviets might defeat Safeguard. The critics claimed, incorrectly, that cost exchange ratios favored the offense by 10:1. That is, it would cost only 10 percent of the defense cost to buy back the needed assured destruction capability.[48]

b. Simple countermeasures could defeat the ground-based ABM missiles. The exo-atmospheric Spartan missile could be defeated with cheap decoys. By detonating a nuclear warhead in space the Soviets could also "black out" the radar so that it couldn't see around the nuclear fireball to guide the interceptors to the nuclear warheads behind the blacked-out region.[49] The endo-atmospheric Sprint, which wouldn't have any problem with decoys (lightweight decoys would burn up as they reentered the atmosphere), could be overwhelmed by putting multiple warheads on the heavy SS-9, that is, increasing the offense capability.[50]

c. Safeguard's computer software would be the most complex ever written. It could never be fully tested and would surely fail.[51] (Watch this one—it returned in the 1980s despite the fact that Safeguard worked well, as discussed in the conclusion.)

d. The system was vulnerable. A Soviet first strike directed at the ABM radars, of which there would be only a small number, could simply and cheaply defeat the whole system.

ABM proponents were inept in countering these arguments—despite the fact that potent counterarguments existed. The primary argument of the proponents was a rehash of Wohlstetter's 1959 strategic concern, the disarming first strike.[52] ABM proponents based their argument on a concern that the Soviet SS-9 ICBM, equipped with MIRVs, could effect a devastating first strike against US land-based missile forces.[53] The critics countered that the United States possessed redundant assured destruction capability in its submarines and surviving land-based bombers and missiles. The proponents were reluctant to admit that our actual deterrent strategy was warfighting. While the quality of a MAD deterrent was little affected by a Soviet first strike, a warfighting deterrent would degrade considerably from such a strike. The proponents therefore lost the argument.

The ABM proponents were ineffective in countering the technical arguments as well. The critics made numerous technical errors. But defense professionals are not comfortable with public arguments of sensitive subjects. They generally avoided taking the critics on. For example, the critics' cost exchange ratio, 10:1 in favor of the offense, was attributed to statements made by Secretary McNamara in 1967. In fact, he had given cost-exchange numbers much closer to 1:1 in his 1967 posture statement.[54] The proponents never publicly challenged this disinformation, which came from much older statements made by McNamara. To the proponents, used to dealing with the public through closed hearings before friendly defense-minded legislators, public debate was alien and inappropriate.

The most devastating blow to the ABM cause was the loss of the moral high ground. By rejecting population defense, the proponents had nothing to offer the public. Without the promise of population defense, the proponents implicitly conceded that nuclear weapons striking the Soviet Union were the basis of deterrence, not the defense of the United States. To an undefended public it was moot whether these targets were a few hundred Soviet cities or a few thousand Soviet military targets.

On 6 August 1969 the Senate approved Safeguard on a tie vote. Vice President Agnew cast the deciding vote. This was a Pyrrhic victory at best—it was the first time that a strategic system supported by an administration and the Congressional Armed Services Committees came close to failure. Within days of the Senate vote, the Soviet Union agreed to arms control negotiations on the ABM issue.[55]

The Triumph of Detente (1972)

When President Johnson agreed in 1967 to let McNamara unleash the arms controllers, US strategic defense was doomed. To be sure, the Soviet change of heart on arms control was complex. Nonetheless, most experts believe Moscow's 1969 about-face was primarily a realization that Safeguard beat out by far the Soviet Galosh as an ABM. Soviet defense lagged at least a decade behind the United States in the late 1960s.[56] The Galosh was similar to, and suffered many of the weaknesses of, the Nike Zeus—abandoned by the United States in 1963.

To the ABM negotiators, it was a dream come true.[57] To these arms controllers, Soviet interest in limiting defense was an implicit acceptance of MAD. The SALT I negotiations, begun in 1969 and destined to last more than two years, culminated in the ABM Treaty and an interim agreement on strategic offensive arms called SALT I.

The United States delegation to the SALT talks clearly believed that they had educated the Soviets into accepting MAD. During the 1972 ABM Treaty ratification hearings, US Chief Negotiator Ambassador Gerard Smith, an outspoken critic of strategic defense in the 1980s, told Senator Jackson:

"I think that the Soviets, as a result of the SALT negotiations, have moved towards accepting the concept of assured destruction."[58]

The administration did not share Smith's enthusiasm for MAD, but pushed the ABM Treaty for different reasons. Secretary of State Henry Kissinger rejected MAD and contradicted Smith on what constituted deterrence in his statement during those same ratification hearings:

> The implications of this [ABM Treaty] are what they have always been over the past five years, because both sides are now vulnerable to each, and therefore, the simplistic notions of the early 1960s which measured deterrent by the amount of civilian carnage that could be inflicted by one side on the other were always wrong; hence, to consider the massive use of nuclear weapons in terms of the destruction of civilian population, one faces a political impossibility, not to speak of a moral impossibility.[59]

Kissinger and other administration testimony revealed the real reason behind the ABM and SALT I Treaties. The MIRV had made ABMs ineffective in a warfighting strategy. The Nixon administration—willing to take risks to shore up its popularity, as the Watergate scandal later showed—needed an arms control deal. The MIRV made this possible. First, Soviet MIRVs would soon be able to defeat Safeguard, and at less cost than it would take to beef up the defense. Second, US MIRVs made it possible to build up our warfighting potential without increasing the total number of missiles. A ban of large-scale defenses and a freeze on missile numbers therefore had little impact on strategic plans. If the arms controllers wanted to pretend that the Soviets had accepted MAD, that was fine. The deal had little strategic impact.

Voices raised against the ABM Treaty were few and barely heard. Some, such as D. G. Brennan, who had spoken for a new strategy based on population defense, saw the Treaty as a foreclosure on that moral alternative.[60] Others, such as Edward Teller, father of the hydrogen bomb, feared that the ABM Treaty would stop research on advanced defensive possibilities, those very possibilities which could address Safeguard's shortcomings. Lasers were one of Teller's possibilities.[61] Some defense-minded senators also objected. Senator Henry Jackson,

Democrat from Washington, worried that arms control, even cosmetic arms control which was based on strategic fantasies like MAD, would damage US security.[62]

While failing to stop the Treaty, the voices of caution won three minor victories. First, Gerard Smith was required to make a unilateral statement to the Soviets that, if arms control following the Treaty did not validate MAD, the ABM Treaty itself would have failed: "If an agreement providing for more complete strategic offensive arms limitations were not achieved within five years, US supreme interests would be jeopardized. Should that occur, it would constitute a basis for withdrawal from the ABM Treaty."[63]

Second, the administration was forced to promise a vigorous research, development, and *deployment* program within the confines of the Treaty.[64] This was to include the allowed deployment of two ABM sites—one to defend the National Command Authority (Washington, DC), the other to defend a Minuteman missile base. A 1974 Protocol to the Treaty lowered the allowed sites for each side to one.[65] Third, US abilities to pursue advanced ABM technologies, particularly lasers, were to be guaranteed.

The provisions for advanced research and development became a major issue in the 1980s, so I will review them here. During the 1972 negotiations the United States sought to prohibit all but basic research on advanced ABM systems.[66] The Soviet Union wanted limits solely on deployments. As usual in arms control, the Soviets won.

To follow the esoteric legal arguments, you must understand several technical distinctions. The ABM Treaty addresses these topics:

1. Allowed ABM systems. These are fixed land-based systems having three specified components: radars, launchers and interceptors. Each side can have no more than 100 interceptors and launchers. The size and location of radars were also limited.

2. Mobile ABM systems. Mobile systems based on land, at sea, in the air or in space, are prohibited from either development or deployment. The Treaty specifies only systems based on the three standard components—radars, launchers, and interceptors.

3. Other Physical Principle (OPP) systems. An agreed statement (Agreed Statement "D") appended to the ABM Treaty specifies that these systems may be developed, but not deployed unless agreed in new negotiations. This statement appears to apply to mobile OPP systems. The mobile systems for which development is prohibited are only those containing the non-OPP radars, launchers and interceptors as components.

During the Treaty negotiations the Soviets allowed the United States to limit category two activities to "research," prohibiting "development." However, the Soviets identified research with their word for "creation," which includes most activities the United States would call "development." The Treaty actually prohibits only system and major component prototype field testing—activities which usually occur as part of US deployment activities rather than development. The Soviet Union had won an agreement which places few, if any, limits on ABM activities short of deployment.

OPP systems were another major area of discussion during the Treaty negotiations. There were specific discussions on two types of systems—those based on lasers and those based on optical sensors.[67] Here, as with definitions of research, the Soviets sought an open-ended agreement. The United States wanted OPP work restricted to laboratories. This argument was not only between the Soviets and the US delegation. Within the US Government the Department of Defense also sought to allow all research, development and testing of OPP systems. The MAD advocates within the Arms Control and Disarmament Agency disagreed. Documents from this period and later show that the Department of Defense prevailed.[68] The Soviets carried the day and Agreed Statement D specified only: "That in the event ABM systems based on other physical principles and including components capable of substituting for ABM interceptor missiles, ABM launchers, or ABM radars are created in the future, specific limitations ... would be subject to discussion...." If the reader doubts that the Soviets considered this "carte blanche," consider Soviet Minister of Defense Andrei A. Grechko's 1972 statement that the Treaty "does not place any limitation on carrying out research and experimental work directed toward solving the problem of defense of the country against nuclear attack."[69]

How have these Soviet "loopholes" in the Treaty been used by the United States? Until 1983 and the SDI, the answer would have been "not at all." Figure 8 shows Soviet and US ballistic missile warhead growth since 1972. The Treaty appears to have had no impact on offensive arsenal growth. Whether one views the arms control process as a success or not, there can be no doubt that Ambassador Smith's unilateral statement was unambiguously breached. Yet, despite the Treaty's absolute failure to usher in mutually assured destruction, strategic theory's advocates hail the Treaty as a great success.[70]

The ink was barely dry on the ABM Treaty when the United States dismantled its allowed ABM system at Grand Forks, North Dakota. More seriously, the United States abandoned ABM research and development. Figure 9 shows what happened to US research and development funding for missile defense during the 1970s. This is scarcely the "robust" program promised during the ABM Treaty hearings.

The OPP system issue demonstrates an even more tangled web. No careful examination of this issue was done by the United States until 1985. The fact that the ABM Treaty negotiators failed to limit the Soviet activities at the negotiation table did not stop them from suggesting to Congress that they had. The 1972 ABM Treaty ratification hearings were themselves a marvel of disinformation on this issue—providing ammunition for both sides in what has become one of the most heated arguments of the 1980s. Since 1985 there has been a thorough review of the ABM Treaty negotiating record by the Department of State which shows that the Soviets had not signed up to what is now known as the "restrictive" interpretation prohibiting development and testing of mobile OPP systems. Statements by the Soviets in subsequent negotiations and deliberations, as well as actual Soviet testing in space of mobile OPP ABM sensors, further show that the Soviets do not accept and are not abiding by the "restrictive" interpretation. This issue had become, by

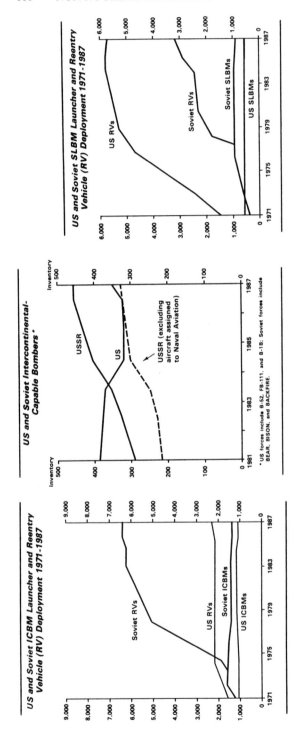

Source: US Department of Defense, *Soviet Military Power 1987* (Washington, DC: US Government Printing Office, 1987), pp. 29, 31, 37.

Figure 8. Growth in the US and Soviet Ballistic Missile Warheads since 1971. Neither country reduced warheads toward a MAD level as mandated by the ABM Treaty.

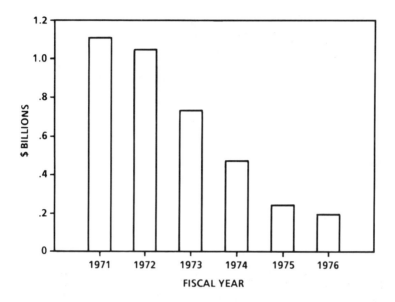

IMPACT OF THE SIGNING OF THE ABM TREATY ON FUNDING
FOR THE ARMY BALLISTIC MISSILE DEFENSE PROGRAM
($ IN MILLIONS)

	1971	1972	1973	1974	1975	1976
PROCUREMENT*	620	599	264	124	2	0
R&D**	490	450	471	351	241	197
TOTAL	1,110	1,049	735	475	243	197

* SENTINEL/SAFEGUARD
** INCLUDES: SAFEGUARD PROGRAM, SYSTEM TECHNOLOGY PROGRAM, AND
ADVANCED TECHNOLOGY PROGRAM.

Figure 9. Impact of the ABM Treaty on Ballistic Missile Defense Research and Development and Procurement. The reduction in funding ran exactly counter to congressional and administration promises.

1986, a contentious political football with those favoring MAD or warfighting deterrent strategies arguing for the restrictive interpretation, while those favoring the "liberal" interpretation supported defense-reliant deterrence. By arguing over legalistic nuances of the Treaty, all concerned were avoiding the central issue of what is the best deterrent strategy for the United States.

The upshot of my discussion here is that the ABM Treaty has turned into a defeat for all three US deterrent schools. It has unfortunately taken on a life of its own. It did not establish

MAD as its US drafters intended, but it resulted in unilateral loss of US ABM research, development and deployment options that its administration backers intended to continue. Finally, and most seriously, it has been taken far beyond its negotiated provisions in an effort to stifle research and development upon which alternate strategies might be based.

Strategic Defense (1983)

The great 1980s debate began with President Reagan's 23 March 1983 speech. The Strategic Defense Initiative, or SDI, was established in January 1984 after several technical and policy studies.[71] SDI critics liked to take President Reagan to task for springing the SDI on an unsuspecting public with little prior analysis or thought. This was not true, however, and the SDI critics knew it.

The SDI had its roots in the ABM Treaty debate. Those who objected to the MAD framework of the Treaty conducted numerous studies during the mid- and late 1970s. The Reagan administration was committed to defense-reliant deterrence from the moment it took office. MAD adherents knew this and published numerous technical and political articles attacking the concept between 1981 and 1983.[72] One finds it hard to believe that they were "surprised" by a program they had anticipated and railed against for years.

In the mid-1970s various strategic analysts, many of them political conservatives, became disturbed with "mirror image" assessments of Soviet intentions. With the signing of the ABM Treaty, many came to assume that MAD was the Soviet strategy as it was ours. In fact, as I have shown, neither side adopted MAD. In 1975, President Ford's Foreign Intelligence Advisory Board commissioned outside studies to provide alternate assessments of Soviet intentions. These were to be "alternate" to CIA estimates which insisted that the Soviets had adopted MAD. The outside study members were designated Team B, headed by Harvard Soviet scholar Richard Pipes. They concluded that the Soviet Union did not accept MAD and was seeking nuclear superiority—in particular, a credible first-strike capability.[73]

A second thread leading to SDI was the Committee on the Present Danger (CPD)—a bipartisan group formed in 1976. CPD included many of the most respected defense professionals of the period. Among its other positions, the CPD opposed the SALT II strategic offensive arms agreements and suggested reconsidering the role of strategic defense. Some key members of CPD and Team B participants became senior officials and advisors to the Reagan administration, and their role in developing the SDI concept is certainly no mystery.[74]

Between 1981 and 1983 the Defense Science Board, the senior Defense Department advisory group, considered strategic defense possibilities in several studies.[75] Three technical developments, widely publicized by enthusiasts of these technologies, generated public pressure for a renewed commitment to strategic defense. First, and by far the most important, was the High Frontier group. Formed in 1980 and headed by former Defense Intelligence Agency head and Team B member Lt. Gen. Daniel Graham, High Frontier conducted technical studies in 1981-1982 on possible strategic defense systems.[76] It concluded that space-based kinetic energy weapons—the equivalent of air-to-air missiles mounted on satellites—could provide an affordable near-term missile defense. Second, in the late 1970s a group of four laser experts convinced many in Washington that space-based lasers could be an effective near-term defense option.[77] Based on their efforts, the Carter administration approved in 1979 a development program to field a space-laser prototype in the early 1990s. Among the converts were Republican Senator Malcolm Wallop of Wyoming and his staff assistant, Angelo Codavilla. These individuals were effective and persuasive advocates of the space laser approach. Third, Edward Teller, father of the hydrogen bomb, publicized work by his protégés at Lawrence Livermore National Laboratories. The Livermore work showed that a laser might be powered with a nuclear explosion. These X-ray lasers could strike ballistic missiles or warheads in space and provide an effective strategic defense.

Despite much information to the contrary, SDI critics love to cite Edward Teller as the SDI source. While his great prestige in Washington and position as an informal advisor to President Reagan certainly made him influential, the fact that he was advocating a nuclear solution to a nuclear problem was not well received by the President.[78]

By 1983, the technical promise of new strategic defense technologies was well known. However, the nuclear freeze provided the key impetus to starting the SDI. The Joint Chiefs of Staff, aware particularly of the High Frontier concept, recognized that their plans were in trouble. The pressure for a nuclear freeze appeared certain to block building the new MX missile in sufficient numbers to recover an effective warfighting deterrent. In early 1983 the Joint Chiefs suggested to the President that the time was ripe to press publicly for the new defensive strategy they knew he favored.[79] Quick studies by Presidential Science Advisor George Keyworth in late 1982 and early 1983 had verified that there was at least one promising technical approach.[80] With all signals go, President Reagan pressed ahead with his famous 23 March 1983 speech. Following technical and policy studies in the summer of 1983, the SDI was formally established in 1984 with the charter to develop the technical basis for a shift to a defense-reliant deterrent strategy.

SDI critics, mostly liberal and members of the scientific community, have tried to replay the 1960s ABM debate. They have had some success in slowing the SDI, but face a much different situation than they had earlier. In the 1960s they were pushing MAD against advocates of nuclear warfighting, in the 1990s they face a much different non-nuclear defensive strategy. There are two crucial aspects to the 1990s debate which profoundly alter it: space and morality.

The idea for space-based defenses first emerged in the Ballistic Missile Boost Intercepts (BAMBI) program started in 1958.[81] Space-based defensive systems make a multilayered defense possible—with the first layer operating almost from the instant an enemy missile lifts off. Whereas the 1950s and 1960s systems could be attacked as "Maginot Lines," multilayered defenses are much different.

History has shown that single-layer defenses—as the 1930s French Maginot Line—fail catastrophically. If breached in a single place or simply gone around, such defenses are worthless. Contrast the Maginot Line with the highly successful British defenses during World War II. The latter had several layers

—the first layer was the British forces in France, the second layer the British Fleet defense of the English Channel, the third layer the Royal Air Force, and the final layer shore defenses and the Home Guard. Taken singly these defenses were relatively weak—the first failed at Dunkirk. As a layered system, however, they were strong enough to deter a major invasion of the British Isles.

The key to effective defense is its ability to operate within most of the battle space through which an aggressor is attacking. If the defense controls—or at least operates effectively—in most of this space, it has a potential advantage. Conversely, if the offense can use most or all of this space to prepare and coordinate its attack, it usually dominates. The missile defenses of the 1950s and 1960s gave up most of the battle space to the offense—for this reason they were likely to fail. By the 1980s, technology had advanced to the point where the BAMBI concept—basically similar to High Frontier's approach—became feasible and affordable.[82] By operating in space, the defense can control most of the battle space. Thus, space operations are the key to effective defenses.

Against the compelling strategic realities of space, SDI critics raised two objections. First, they charged that space defenses would be vulnerable and could be cheaply negated.[83] As I discuss in the conclusion, this argument is not supported by technical facts. Second, following Soviet propaganda, some SDI critics worried over the "militarization" of space. This charge ignores the fact that it was the ICBM which not only militarized space but *nuclearized* it as well. When the first German V-2 broke through the edges of space, that medium was forever broached. In addition to raising the possibility of attack through space, ICBMs have also been the basis of launch vehicles since the 1950s. In the 1980s, 60 percent of long-haul military communications go through space systems and most surveillance is space-based.[84] Space has long since been militarized; it is not SDI which raises this problem.

More significant than technical manifest destiny is the moral dimension of the SDI. President Reagan's March 1983 speech said it clearly: "What if free people could live secure in the knowledge that their security did not rest upon the threat of

instant retaliation to deter a Soviet attack?'' The key point of the
Reagan administration is that defenses are designed to protect
people. Senior administration officials constantly stress this
point. For example:

> It is not our missiles we seek to protect but our people, and
> we must never lose sight of that goal.[85]
>
> > Caspar Weinberger, 1 July 1986
> > Secretary of Defense

> Protecting weapons represents no change in present policy.
> It simply strengthens—entrenches—a de facto doctrine of
> Mutual Assured Destruction. Protecting people, on the
> other hand, holds out the promise of dramatic change. The
> clear purpose of the President has been repeated time and
> time again.[86]
>
> > George Keyworth, 21 May 1985
> > Science Advisor to the President

Morality was a strong rationale underlying the military's push
for SDI. Admiral James Watkins, Chief of Naval Operations in
the mid–1980s, was central in his support of the SDI. Moral
supremacy of a defense-reliant deterrent played a strong role in
his thinking.[87]

Morality in US deterrent strategy goes well on Main Street
too. In the early 1980s the ''nuclear freeze''—a cessation of all
nuclear weapons development, testing, and production—was
extremely popular. As a response to that movement, the SDI
was singularly successful. Although the freeze started as a grass
roots movement with overwhelming public support, the SDI
quickly banished it from center stage. The concept of defense-
reliant deterrence holds overwhelming public support—
consistently above 50 percent and frequently as high as 80
percent.[88]

The moral argument was not greeted with enthusiasm by
advocates of alternate strategies—a tribute to its effectiveness.
In fact, it gave them fits. Consider a few quotes from SDI
critics:

> Until there are inventions that have not even been imag-
> ined, a defense robust and cheap enough to replace deter-
> rence will remain a pipe dream. Emotional appeals that

defense is morally superior to deterrence are therefore "pernicious."[89]

> Robert McNamara and Hans Bethe
> July 1985

Cries of the immorality of deterrence are both premature and pernicious.[90]

> James Schlesinger
> 24 October 1984

In the lexicons of both MAD and nuclear warfighting advocates it appears that the word "pernicious" must be redefined as "effective."

The "pernicious" moral argument has also disturbed US allies. Conservative European government officials and strategists know that the moral argument is effective. They also stress that it plays into the hands of leftists who believe there is nothing to deter. Consequently, advocates of the current warfighting strategy and European flexible response approaches have sought to modify the moral argument.[91]

Requirements of a Non-Nuclear Deterrence

SDI critics translate the advocate's statements about defending people into something much different, and they insist that the advocates want to replace deterrence. To do so, the critics assert, requires perfect defenses. This specious argument ignores the two sides of the deterrence coin. On the one side, deterrence works because an aggressor fears punishment, while on the other side deterrence works if the aggressor fears his military efforts will be denied. A child told to stay out of the cookie jar might be deterred either by the threat of a spanking or by the fact that the cookie jar has been clearly placed outside his reach.

Denying Soviet War Aims

In chapter 1, I described how MAD is pure punishment deterrence. Retaliation-based warfighting strategies have elements of both punishment and denial. Inasmuch as the retaliation smashes Soviet military power, it denies them the instruments of success. But since it also could destroy Soviet leadership and economic infrastructure, it has elements of punishment as well. Defense-reliant deterrence is pure denial, in contrast.

The Soviet Union understands these distinctions. The Russian language has two words for deterrence—one translates as "holding back," the other as "intimidation."[92] When the United States speaks of deterrence, the Soviets always translate it into "intimidation." Some believe that this stark representation of US strategic policy is the root of many of our difficulties with the Soviets.[93]

If we are to deny Soviet war aims, we must understand what they are. While Soviet offensive forces are a major instrument of their policy, I believe that some US experts are mistaken in regarding it as the sole instrument. This is another case of "mirror imaging." Since we rely almost exclusively on offensive nuclear forces, we assume our adversary does as well. SDI's focus on only the Soviet offensive nuclear forces is its major failing. As constituted, the SDI is developing means to deny only the war aims of the Soviet nuclear offensive arm—the Strategic Rocket Troops. A coherent US strategy must address all elements of Soviet power, particularly their political initiatives and formidable ground forces.

In this section, I restrict myself to the goal of the SDI as constituted—to deny the mission of the Strategic Rocket Troops. These Soviet forces have the mission of destroying several thousand military targets in the West.

Whatever the Strategic Rocket Troops' mission, they must have some target "set" to destroy. Soviet leaders must require, as do their US counterparts, a minimum percentage of that set be destroyed. For the purpose of my example, let's assume that number is 800 out of a target set of 1000.

Suppose that the United States builds a defense with 3 layers. Our number of layers is thus $L = 3$. The layers aren't perfect—they "leak" some warheads through. If each layer leaks 20 percent of those it faces, then leakage for each layer is, $E = 0.2$. The overall system of three leaky layers has an effectiveness of:

$$A = 1 - E^L$$

In our example of three 20 percent leaky layers, the system would have an effectiveness of 0.992—in other words it would stop 99.2 percent of the warheads fired at the United States.

Let's turn the problem around and look at it from a Soviet targeteer's viewpoint. He can't know which warheads will get through to which targets—he just knows that 99.2 percent of what he fires will be stopped. He can only consider the problem from a statistical viewpoint—on the average he can guess how many warheads will get through to a given target.

For a given target, the probability of getting a single warhead through is:

$$PD = 1 - A^W$$

In our example with $A = 0.992$, let's assume the Soviets fire 100 warheads at the target, so $W = 100$. Their statistical probability of getting one warhead through is $PD = 0.56$ or 56 percent—a lot of warheads for an uncertain result.

Let's now turn to an example where the Soviets need to destroy 800 out of 1000 targets. If the Soviets have no preference concerning the targets, we can treat each target the same and get $PD = 0.8$, assuming that firing at 1000 targets with an 80 percent probability to hit each one, will result in 800 being destroyed. To have an 80 percent confidence in striking one target, the Soviets would need the following number of warheads:

$$W = \frac{\log(1\text{-PD})}{\log (A)}$$

To figure how many warheads are needed to hit all 800 required targets, T, let's multiply by the number of potential targets, M $= 1000$.

$$T = \frac{\log(1 - PD) \times M}{\log(1 - E^L)}$$

In our example, the Soviets would need almost 200,000 warheads to hit 80 percent of their 1,000 targets. Moreover, nuclear warheads are unreliable. It's reasonable to assume 50 percent reliability per warhead, so the Soviets might have to plan on getting two or three warheads through to ensure their required success rate.[94]

In figure 10 I show some results of these calculations for defensive systems with one, two and three layers—each layer

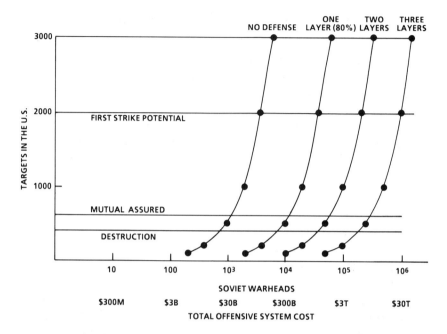

Source: US Department of Defense, Strategic Defense Initiative Organization.

Figure 10. Effects of Layered Defenses on Soviet Targeting. With a requirement for two warheads per target and no defenses, today's Soviet arsenal is way oversized for MAD, but optimally sized for attacks on US military forces. The addition of a single 80% effective defense layer would complicate Soviet strategy—but not prevent the Soviets from staying with it. A two-layer defense, with each layer 80% effective, would prevent the Soviets from maintaining a warfighting strategy. A three-layer defense would even deny a MAD strategy. Soviet costs to add warheads are based on MX costs of $20 million per warhead. The two- and three-layer defenses would easily drive the Soviets to unaffordable expenditures.

having a 20 percent leakage. I also assume that the Soviets must get two warheads through the defense to kill one target.

These curves show that even against modest one- and two-layer defenses the Soviets would need hundreds of thousands of warheads to destroy any reasonable fraction of US military targets. We can use this same analysis to study other target bases, such as a city-busting MAD target set. Against a three-layered defense the current Soviet offensive arsenal would be able to hit only 30 cities. That would kill millions, but would not represent assured destruction as it has been defined for the past three decades.

In 1984, after the SDI program got under way, it came under especially heavy criticism for inconsistency. Government officials had made many statements about the program's goals—often the speakers had only a passing familiarity with the program and with deterrent strategy. The Arms Control Organization, consisting largely of MAD adherents, was able to compile 26 pages of conflicting statements on SDI's strategic goals.[95] For this reason, the Administration moved to clarify the goals and published in January 1985 a pamphlet entitled *The President's Strategic Defense Initiative*.[96] It specified three requirements for an effective defense:

> 1. They [defenses] must, at a minimum, be able to destroy a sufficient portion of an aggressor's attacking forces to deny him confidence in the outcome of an attack or deny an aggressor the ability to destroy a militarily significant portion of the target base he wished to attack.

> 2. Any effective defense must, of course, be survivable.... The defense system need not be invulnerable, but must be able to maintain a sufficient degree of effectiveness to fulfill its mission, even in the face of determined attacks against it.

> 3. The defensive system must be able to maintain its effectiveness against the offense at less cost than it would take to develop offensive countermeasures and proliferate the ballistic missiles necessary to overcome it.

These three criteria were ignored until Paul Nitze, a man with impeccable arms control credentials, repeated them some months later.[97] They became known as the three Nitze Criteria:

effectiveness, survivability, and cost-effectiveness at the margin, and were enshrined in a Presidential directive promulgated in the summer of 1985,[98] which also included an NSC-enforced "gag" order to ensure compliance.

We have discussed what "effective" means in this section. In the next few paragraphs I will define what we must do to meet the other two criteria. (In the conclusion, I will discuss how possible defensive systems can meet these requirements in the 1990s and beyond.)

Would the Soviets sit still as their trillion-dollar offensive forces are rendered "impotent and obsolete?" Faced with a defense that negates their missile force, they would consider one of the following alternatives:

1. Build enough new missiles to recover their original damage capability.

2. Build a capability to attack and destroy enough of the defense (defense "suppression") to recover their original strategy.

3. Find other ways to accomplish their strategic goals— new offensive systems or different types of offensive systems.

4. Develop alternate strategic objectives.

To succeed in its role, a defense-reliant approach must close off each alternative. The Soviets might not fully accept capitalist figures of merit—i.e., how much it costs. But neither can they ignore costs. We shall thus consider strategic requirements in terms of the economic figures of merit favored by Western strategists.

What does "cost effective at the margin" mean? SDI critics quickly seized on a one-for-one trade. The Union of Concerned Scientists translates this Nitze criterion into: "It should cost less for the United States to shoot down a Soviet missile than for the USSR to build that additional missile."[99] There was a major tempest in a teapot during 1986 when Defense Secretary Weinberger objected to this way of considering the criterion. The compromise between the State and Defense Departments on this issue was a masterpiece in noninformation.[100]

In the previous section we defined defense effectiveness in terms of Soviet offensive strategy. If the Soviet strategy requires 2000 US targets to be destroyed, and we can limit them to a small faction of these, that is "effective." Cost-effectiveness at the margin follows directly. If the Soviets respond to an initial US defense by adding enough offensive forces to bring them back to confidence in destroying the original 2000 targets, that will cost them some large amount. The United States might respond with an improved defense—costing some other amount. The defense need only be beefed up enough to once again deny Soviet objectives. If the Soviet offensive response costs more than the US defensive counter—that is cost-effective at the margin.

Let's consider an example. Suppose the United States builds a two-layer defense with 20 percent leakage per layer. We shall assume initial Soviet strategy required 2000 targets destroyed. With their current force, the new US defense would lower them to only 100 targets. At first, as they add warheads, they must add lots for each additional target they get. Figure 10 (p. 120) shows that they could double the number and only add a few hundred targets. But at some point the defense will be saturated and each additional warhead will get through the defense to its target. Suppose the Soviets could get back to their initial state by adding 15,000 warheads—costing them the equivalent of $300 billion. If we can build up our defense so it once again denies Soviet *targeting* objectives for less than $300 billion— then our move is cost-effective at the margin. Because of the statistical uncertainty which defenses introduce, they enjoy far better than a one-to-one leverage on the offense. This is one of the advantages to a defense-reliant approach.

Survivability is similar to cost effectiveness at the margin. The Soviets might, as they have threatened to do,[101] try to shoot down a system rather than overwhelm it. The anti-satellites, if that be their choice, would cost them some amount. Moreover, this defense suppression must be good enough to get them back to the point where they were before the defenses went up. The United States could then respond, either with survivability enhancements or simply by proliferating the defenses so they could accomplish their mission despite losses. If the US response costs less than the Soviet defense suppression, the defensive system will have met the survivability requirement.

The Soviets have another option; they could build a totally new type of offensive system. It might rely on offensive missiles which slip by the defense, or a non-ballistic approach such as cruise missiles. Whatever their response, it will cost and it must be good enough to preserve their strategy. For the United States there will be new defensive means to counter the Soviet countermeasures. If these defensive moves cost less than the Soviet offensive countermeasures, the defense wins.

Of course, the Soviets might try a combination of more offense, defense suppression, and new offensive systems. No matter, if the defense can prevent Soviet mission accomplishment more cheaply—we have the defense-dominant situation we seek.

What if the Soviets change their requirements and not their systems? Suppose they adopt a new strategy requiring fewer targets for success. Suppose, even, that they adopt MAD as McNamara and others assert they have.[102] While I believe, as I will show in the next chapter, that the Soviets will never voluntarily move away from an offensive warfighting strategy, we must consider the possibility that they will. If that happens, we must have in hand defenses which can deny the new Soviet strategy and meet the same criteria we have today. This brings us to the next objective—assured survival.

Assured Survival

Defining assured survival is harder than defining assured destruction. Whatever its definition, many believe it to be the only legitimate goal for SDI.[103] To this point deterrence is only a means to prevent war. MAD prevents war by threatening mass death to the enemy population, while warfighting deters by threatening the destruction of an aggressor's armed might. Defense-reliant deterrence works when the enemy's forces are militarily impotent. But when we consider assured survival we have shifted to the question of damage limitation after deterrence fails.

In the 1960s, the United States worried about how to limit damage if deterrence failed, but these requirements conflicted with MAD. MAD adherents solved the problem by insisting that deterrence cannot fail, so we don't need to worry about damage limiting. Warfighters knew what to do if deterrence failed—win the war! But winning wars might have little to do with assuring survival, since all too often in war the village must be destroyed to "save" it.

Unlike MAD and warfighting approaches, defense-reliant deterrence is consistent with damage limitation, and ultimately assured survival. Assured survival means having our survival in our own hands rather than in someone else's. But we know that Soviet ability to destroy 1000 targets is less "survival" for the United States than if they can only get 100 US targets. While a single warhead falling on a nation does not mean its destruction, as World War II's end proved, zero damage must be our ultimate goal. Unlike other forms of deterrence, every increase in assured survival is also an increase in defensive deterrence. If limiting the Soviets to 1000 warheads getting through provides some defensive deterrence, limiting them to 100 provides better deterrence and better damage limitation. Our objective, therefore, should be to establish a trend where every increase in deterrence also results in increased survival should deterrence fail. We will reach assured survival in discrete steps—not in a giant leap.

Transition Stability

If at any time the march toward assured survival raises the pressures for war, the transition is said to be "unstable." The unstable transition to defense-reliant deterrence is a favorite theme of SDI critics and even some advocates. As I showed in chapter 2, it is Glenn Kent's diagram with its overlapping areas of "conditional survival" which cause this problem. I believe this "instability" is a red herring. The problem is that Kent's charts are strategy blind and zero-point unstable.

What do I mean by "strategy blind"? Quite simply, the conditional survival "problem" ignores the concept of strategic victory at the base of both Soviet and US strategies. The alleged instability results when a side strikes first for fear the other will preempt it. This scenario ignores the fact that both the United States and the Soviet Union have a strategic target base numbering in the thousands. The decision to strike depends on whether that strike can meet its strategic damage objectives—not on whether a side thinks it can get more warheads through if it strikes now rather than waiting. If one side strikes first and only destroys a few of the other side's targets, it may be that the retaliation will be more "ragged" but neither country will have fatally damaged the other's warfighting abilities. A single falling warhead does not make the difference between victory and defeat. Conversely, defenses always lower the possibility of victory for the aggressor. Their presence on both sides decreases both the incentives for going first (the possibility of gaining a strategic victory) and pressures for going first (the fear the opponent will gain victory by going first).

What do I mean by zero-point unstable? This fake instability occurs when zero damage is inserted on Kent's transition chart (figure 7, p. 88). As any mathematician knows, calculations containing zero in them are often unstable. The alleged instability happens when defenses have gotten good enough so that one side could get only a few warheads through the other's defense. This attack might destroy enough of the victim's warheads so that his retaliation cannot get back through the aggressor's defense. The side which preempted would thus suffer no damage, but the victim would have taken some nuclear hits. As I discussed in chapter 1, it is not possible to assure zero damage to a country with any kind of defenses. But more to the point, when the damage is so small, even to the victim, the military gains are so marginal, and the uncertainty so high that the complicated stability criteria of MAD and warfighting strategies lose their meaning.

These "instabilities" both ignore strategy. If a first or preemptive strike had little impact on the war's outcome, the situation would be much different than today. The incentives and pressures for a "Pearl Harbor-type" attack only exist when that attack could mean the difference between victory or defeat. Today, a first strike could well mean the difference between military victory and defeat—and that is unstable. But when a first strike will get only a handful of warheads through the defenses the problem disappears. Regardless of details, the situation would be more stable than today's circumstances.

If the defenses, during deployment, are especially vulnerable to suppression, they could be a tempting target. If one side sees the other deploying a defense which could put him at a disadvantage, he might think of removing it while the defense is still vulnerable. Further, it might not cost the aggressor much to remove the defenses at this point. In the conclusion, I show that the types which would be deployed do not present an opportunity for this easy type of defense suppression.

Another type of transition instability exists. Its proposers grant that a strategic defense might be effective. But they fear that the Soviets, aware that their trillion-dollar investment might soon be useless, would use their defense before it was destroyed. This argument ignores several items. First, defenses will not go in overnight—so General Secretary Gorbachev won't wake up one morning with a sudden decision on his hands. Second, the United States is proposing a cooperative transition where *no one* will have an advantage which would scare the other one into a rash act. Third, the Soviets are already installing their own defenses, so they have little worry about being left behind. Finally, the Soviet Union is a profoundly conservative society, as I discuss in the next chapter. It simply wouldn't risk everything because things looked bleak in the short term—one mustn't forget that the current US deterrent will remain quite capable of destroying the Soviet military as a fighting force until a considerable defense is in place on both sides. The present deterrent will continue to deter even as the defensive component strengthens.

Let us add a final point about transitions before we leave the subject. In the 1960s, the United States moved away from a mixed offensive and defensive force deterrent. As it came to rely more on missiles, for which we didn't have a defense, we dismantled our substantial air defenses. This occurred over the space of a few short years. Yet no one claims that it was particularly unstable. A switch back to greater, and ultimately dominant, reliance on defenses has no features fundamentally different from the 1960s transition—and therefore is likely to be no more unstable.

The Moral Dimension to Strategic Defense

New weapons are frequently regarded as immoral—particularly by those whose military careers are based on old methods and weapons.

> O' curs'd device! base implement of death.
> Fram'd in the Black Tartarean realms beneath!
> By Beelzebub's malicious art design'd
> To ruin all the race of human kind.[104]
>
> Ariosto (1473-1533)

Although Ariosto, a Renaissance warrior, wrote his feelings about gunpowder, they could equally well apply to 20th century "gifts" to mankind such as chemical and nuclear weapons. Over the several thousand years of recorded thought much pondering has gone into the question of morality and war.

Some concepts have stood the test of time. War becomes moral if it meets two criteria. First, it must have limited objectives and be limited in scope. Second, it must involve only professional soldiers who possess a sense of professional ethics. History allows only one exception. The gloves come off if war is waged against "non-humans." Entry into the latter category is earned in a variety of ways—cultural, religious, and moral.

The ancient Greeks had strict limitations to war—a most honorable process restricted to the best elements of society. Wars were to have just causes, there were prohibitions on enslaving the defeated, and there were edicts against civilian destruction. Of course, there were no limitations on action against "non-humans"—i.e., non-Greeks.[105]

In the Middle Ages, the concept of "just war" emerged. Following the teachings of St. Ambrose and St. Augustine, Christian leaders had the right and the responsibility of resisting evil with force. Just war doctrine had two precepts—a just cause and proportionate punishment. The ends must be proportionate to the means. War must be waged for a better peace.[106]

How is a "just" cause determined? No one goes to war for what he believes to be "unjust" reasons. This is the reason for restricting war to proportionate means. To the medieval

Christian war was a trial by combat. In deciding the victor, God decided who was in the right.

Western moral tradition thus places twin constraints on war—honorable and professional soldiers and limited wars.

What of technology, since it would seem that advancing technology violates morality? Technology allows amateurs to engage in war and it raises destruction to levels where noncombatant involvement is inevitable, and so it is that, applied to warfare, it has often been regarded as immoral. The Romans harnessed technology and barbarized warfare. Precision training and technical innovations such as catapults changed war from a contest of valor to "organized bloody drills."[107] The Second Lateran Council of AD 1139 outlawed weapons such as crossbows and siege machines (except for use against non-Christians). The diatribes of the 15th and 16th centuries against gunpowder—an example of which is Ariosto's at the beginning of this section—were based in part on the fact that peasants could use gunpowder to equalize their status against honorable professional soldiers.

Despite history's judgment that technological innovations are immoral, new military inventions have always been used. How is this so? The answer lies in the exceptions granted, for example, in AD 1139. Immoral weapons such as crossbows could always be used against "non-humans." It was easy to define those non-Christians in possession of the Holy Land as "non-humans." Similarly, the religious wars of the 16th and 17th centuries (1562-1648) allowed the unconstrained use of gunpowder against civilians—resulting in the depopulation of Germany during the Thirty Years' War. Once again, religion succeeded in designating the enemy as "non-human." Immoral weapons and practices are always acceptable against them.

The 19th and 20th centuries have not changed things. Total war, using all available technical means, is moral only against an indisputably "non-human" enemy. Only the means of becoming non-human have changed in the past millennia. Ideas are now more capable of rendering a society "non-human" than is religion. The Napoleonic wars became total wars over a clash of ideas, not religion.

World War II was an interesting case. The Allies bombed German cities, confident in the inhumanity of the German people. The Nazi death camps, discovered after the war, only fixed morality on the side of the Allies. The "inhuman" attack on Pearl Harbor earned the Japanese this dubious status. Our atomic bomb retaliation thus became a just retribution. It was only upon reflection that the argument that the bombs saved millions of lives came to the fore.

What of morality and the three deterrent strategies? In the 1950s there was only the faintest whisper of moral concern over US strategy. The reason was that the Soviet Union was understood to be a "godless communist dictatorship," non-human in every respect. This certitude has now changed, and for two reasons. First, the Soviet Government has tried to put on a human face. It's awfully hard to designate a nation as inhuman which sends a magnificent Bolshoi Ballet to visit. Similarly, Soviet arms control negotiators love to present their Western counterparts with humanizing gifts.[108] Second, and more significant, Soviet nuclear arsenals have raised a moral dilemma. While a Western strike against the Soviet Union might kill largely "godless communists," their retaliation would kill many moral Westerners—thus a moral act would inevitably have immoral consequences.

The intrinsic immorality of mass destruction has led to a new morality. As I discussed in chapter 1, the widespread view that nuclear war would end mankind has had a profound impact on moral thought. Freeman Dyson's 1984 book, *Weapons and Hope*, and Jonathan Schell's works, *The Fate of the Earth* (1982) and *The Abolition* (1985), made it clear that the end of the world always qualifies as immoral—as did the Catholic bishops' 1983 Pastoral letter.[109]

The Catholic bishops reaffirmed the 1500-year-old "just war" tradition. But to be just a war must be: (1) the last resort, (2) likely to succeed in its aims, and (3) proportional in the sense that its costs in lives and property justify the gains.

Is Mutually Assured Destruction moral? Inasmuch as the consequences of deterrence failing are mass death and mayhem, the answer must be a firm no. The Catholic bishops and others increasingly reject MAD on this basis. Against this principled onslaught MAD advocates can only assert that deterrence will not fail. They argue that MAD is a fact of life which only arms control can treat, and that is the only moral shield for MAD advocates.

What of nuclear warfighting? On the surface it would seem that this is a more moral strategy. After all, it is directed against military forces, not civilians. As such it seems to meet the ancient criterion of a contest between professional soldiers. Further, flexible response strategies envisage limited objectives and tactics. Yet, nuclear warfighting is even more condemned by religious and secular philosophers.[110] The reason? No one can say that a nuclear war, even restricted to military targets, would not kill millions of non-combatants. Where nuclear warfighting loses out is in its implicit assumption that deterrence could fail. Since it accepts the possibility of megadeaths, although claiming it is more effective in deterring such eventualities, it is considered worse that MAD. Its only weak response is to try to resurrect a ''non-human'' Soviet enemy—a task at which it has been unsuccessful.

What of defense-reliant deterrence? Freeman Dyson advocated defensive strategies as a moral transition from MAD to a non-militarized world. The Catholic bishops seemed to support this idea:

> We do not perceive any situation in which the deliberate initiation of nuclear warfare in however restricted a scale can be morally justified. Non-nuclear attacks by another state must be resisted by other than nuclear means. Therefore, a serious moral obligation exists to develop non-nuclear defensive strategies as rapidly as possible.[111]

Yet, few religious philosophers or other moralists have stepped forward to endorse SDI. Indeed, the Methodist bishops specifically condemned it.[112] Why? I believe the answer is twofold. First, the MAD advocates assert that the transition to a defense-reliant strategy will raise the risk of nuclear war. As I discussed in this chapter, these arguments are controversial at best, and most likely wrong. But there is a second, unfortunate reason why intellectuals oppose SDI. The SDI program was proposed by a conservative Republican president. It has been enthusiastically pushed by the right wing of American politics.

Those most prominent in touting the immorality of nuclear war firmly occupy the left end of American political life. One could hardly expect them to endorse a strategy espoused by a conservative president and political segment they find morally repugnant on every other ground.

As a result, we are confronted by a real dilemma in seeking a strategic consensus. Most Americans find all nuclear strategies immoral: the popularity of the nuclear freeze movement in the early 1980s was testimony to that. Yet, the only alternate strategy—one which is consistent with more than 1000 years of just war tradition—is unacceptable to the political left. It is unacceptable not because of its content, but because of the strange bedfellows which its acceptance would mean. Unless this dilemma is solved, no consensus is possible on either strategic or moral grounds.

4. DISARMAMENT: A NON-DETERRENT STRATEGY

Therefore, determine the enemy's plan and you will know which strategy will be successful and which not.[1]

Sun Tzu
400 BC

I cannot forecast to you the action of Russia. It is a riddle wrapped in a mystery inside an enigma.[2]

Winston Churchill
AD 1939

The Soviet Union—a strange place, a strange people, and a strange government. Like most Americans I knew little about the Soviets. As a member of a US arms control team I sat across a table from them for a year and a half. So much talk of peace and disarmament! (But so much murder and mayhem in the world at Soviet hands as well.[3]) As we talked, 1000 new nuclear warheads poured out of Soviet arsenals. Why? What was their purpose?

There is no doubt that the Strategic Defense Initiative (SDI) has Soviet attention—perhaps as no other event since August 1945. General Secretary Gorbachev has not given a major speech since he took the Soviet helm in which he has not decried US "militarization of space." An unprecedented stream of full color, glossy Soviet publications—many which would put even Madison Avenue to shame—"prove" that SDI will not work, will end arms control, will cause World War III, will escalate the arms race, and will generally be the biggest evil to hit the world since the beginning of time.[4] Troops of no-longer-poorly-dressed propagandists from the Soviet USA/Canada Institute appear more often at US and Western European forums to attack SDI than US officials do to defend it.[5]

133

Western differences with Soviet ideas start with the definition of "strategy." The United States, in particular, considers strategy in its purely military implications. "Strategy" is the big military picture—how we intend to use our forces to win our objectives. "Tactics" is military engineering—how military leaders get each job done. The Soviet Union has three different military concepts. They use the same words for two of their three concepts, "strategy" and "tactics," but the meanings are much different than in the West. Soviet "strategy" is a combination of military and political approaches. United States traditions of separating military and political spheres make this an alien marriage. An explicit definition of strategy was given by Stalin in 1923: "The most important task of strategy is the determination of the basic direction along which the movement of the working class must go, and along which it is most favorable for the proletariat to deliver the main blow to the opponent for the realization of those ends set by the program."[6] What we call strategy—the strictly military big picture—the Soviets identify as their third, intermediate category, "operational art."

Soviet strategy's central theme is political—not military. Marxist-Leninist doctrine teaches that all wars have their roots in class struggle. More to the point, the proletariat—represented by the Soviet leadership—is destined to win. Lenin was particularly fond of Karl von Clausewitz, the father of the political theory of war. Of his famous passage, "War is nothing but the continuation of policy with other means,"[7] Lenin wrote in 1915: "War is the continuation of politics by other (namely violent) means. That well known quotation belongs to one of the deepest writers on military affairs, Clausewitz. Marxists have always considered that thesis the theoretical basis of views on the significance of any given war. Marx and Engels always looked at different wars especially from that point of view."[8]

The thing to remember here is not the words of Lenin or Clausewitz. The converse—politics as a form of war—is what matters to the Soviets.

What are the principal elements of Soviet political warfare? For the purposes of this chapter I identify three.

1. Without a doubt, the primary objective of Soviet strategy *is* peace. There is no hidden Machiavellian meaning here.

Since 1918 Soviet policy and action have been directed toward one thing—peace. Why? In their view peace allows the superior Soviet system to mature and win by non-violent means. Marxist theory arms its adherents with infallable "scientific" tools for using non-violent means to further their struggle. War—particularly high-technology war—threatens to destroy all Marxist gains. The reason is that war is unpredictable. "Scientific" political gains made in war can be overturned by Clausewitz's other concept—"friction"—a term meaning that nothing can be accurately predicted in the fog of war. Consequently, it is precisely in violent struggle where the superiority of Marxist "scientific" analysis and prediction of events are at their least predictable.

We would also do well to remember another Soviet reason for wanting peace. Lenin commented on another Clausewitz quote—"The aggressor is always peace-loving (as Bonaparte always claimed to be); he would prefer to take over our country unopposed"[9]—with the following quip: "Ha Ha—pretty smart."[10]

2. Soviet military doctrine is based on the offensive. If its peace efforts fail, the Soviet Union's armed forces are ready to take the offensive and to win. This approach is not inconsistent with their peace policy, since the Soviets firmly believe that war, if it comes, will be initiated by the West.

Defenses play a role in Soviet offensive strategy—albeit a secondary one. Following Lenin's dictum, "one step back—two steps forward," defensive actions are designed to buy time in order to prepare for a crushing offensive blow.[11] As I discussed in chapter 2, this concept is consistent with US warfighting strategy and with Clausewitz, both of which hold defenses useful only as a means for protecting and preparing for an offensive. With this perspective, the Soviets invariably see the US SDI as an offensive move.

3. It is all to the good if the rules of the game can be frozen. The almost rabid Soviet opposition to the SDI is not based on the role of defenses in deterrent strategies. Quite simply, the Soviets want the United States out of space—as they would any new area that could mean an end run by their adversaries. Space introduces a dramatic and decisive new factor, as did US introduction of nuclear weapons in 1945. The Soviet Union would gladly agree to ban any and all new means of conflict.

Soviet objection to new forms of combat has as much to do with national character as with Marxist theory. The Soviets prefer to play chess, as did their forefathers. They want the rules narrowed and frozen. Confident of their "scientific" approach and the stability of their centrally controlled state, they are sure they will win as long as the rules stay put.

Western states, and the United States in particular, are poker players. American leaders are usually amateurs likely to do best in a fast-paced situation involving frequent new factors. The Soviets know and fear this. Their top objective is therefore peace—and peace arranged such that new factors are unlikely. It is no wonder they came to the 1980s negotiating table at Geneva with such alarm. Expecting to set up the same old arms control chessboard—they saw instead a smiling Uncle Sam riffling his deck of cards and ready for a fast-paced poker hand: "Read 'em and weep—lasers are wild this week!"

Development of Soviet Strategy

Although it is easy to overstate historical impacts on a nation's strategy, we shouldn't ignore these influences. While I cannot attribute Soviet preoccupation with the militarization of space to Catherine the Great's notorious love affairs, the Tsarist period played a critical role in setting current Soviet military strategy. It is instructive to remember that Alexis de Tocqueville predicted in the 18th century that the United States and Russia would become hostile superpowers. He based his conclusion on the two nations' unequaled natural wealth and on their fundamentally different views about human freedoms.[12]

A controversial, although I believe instructive, treatise on the Tsarist roots of modern Soviet behavior is Richard Pipes' *Russia Under the Old Regime*.[13] Several features of current Soviet military strategy emerge from the Tsarist years:

   1. Innate conservatism. Russian agriculture, due to its far northern location, was inherently subsistence farming, and there was little room for mistakes.[14] Mistakes flow from risky initiatives, making initiative bad. Russian and Soviet military literature correspondingly show great distaste for "adventurist" Western approaches.

2. *Rigid central control.* By the 16th century the person in charge had established that he "owned" everything, including the people. In this context it's interesting to note that the Russian word for sovereign means "owner of slaves."[15] The principle of a paternalistic system of central control was well established centuries before the Bolsheviks took power. Soviet strategy emphasizes the virtues of top-down control.[16]

3. *Large, offensively oriented military.* Partly as a result of the need for better land, and partly as a result of a paranoid view of the world, Russia has always been a militarized state. I use the word "paranoid" because Russia has not been successfully overrun since the Mongol invasion of 1236 and has only been seriously threatened twice in the past two centuries—by Napoleon and by Hitler. As an example of extreme militarism, Peter the Great spent two-thirds of the Russian economy on the military—three times the normal rate in Europe at the time.[17]

The Western liberal press has written countless volumes on change in the Soviet Union since Gorbachev became the "owner" of that nation. Some observers in the West are enthralled by his seeming reasonableness.[18] By way of a caution, I must point out that he represents a long line of Russian "reformers" in the tradition of Peter the Great. Tsar Peter was no more interested in a free society than, apparently, is Gorbachev. But Peter noted that his troops did poorly against Western forces because they had failed to keep up with Western technological changes. In Richard Pipes's words, "Peter was interested in power, especially military power, not in Westernization." In Peter's own words, "We need Europe for a few decades, and then we will turn our back on it."[19] It is significant that the Soviets attribute to him the foundations of their art of war.[20]

When the Bolsheviks took over in 1917, drastic changes took place in some elements of Russian society—but not in military strategy. For example, the Bolsheviks kept many Tsarist generals. Indeed, many of these survived the purges of the 1930s to forge the Soviet victory in World War II.[21]

The Bolsheviks added two simple principles to the old Russian strategy. First, they touted the Clausewitzian dictum of war as politics. Second, they regarded their strategy as a manifestation of a superior Marxist/Leninist approach; that is, careful calculations of the "correlation of forces" (COF). COF is similar in some respects to what the United States calls "net assessment." But since the Soviet version includes dynamic as well as static elements, long-term trends must be included in any analysis.[22] Specifically, the Soviets believe that they can quantify, in precise mathematical terms, the factors bearing on a military situation. From these calculations a military leader should be able to decide whether to attack, retreat, play for time, or make some other decisions. This quantitative approach contrasts with "adventuristic" Western strategies such as the German World War II Blitzkrieg or current US deterrent strategies which rely on unquantifiable factors.[23]

The Russian Civil War (1918-1922) and the Great Patriotic War (1941-1945) set Soviet pre-nuclear strategy. Modern Soviet nuclear strategy builds on this base and does not reject it. Of course, Western strategy has also built on a historical base. As I showed in chapter 2, current US nuclear strategy still follows the Douhet strategic aviation doctrines of World War II—but is much less tied to the historical precedents than are the Soviets.

The fundamental Soviet warfighting principle is the offensive.[24] But what do I mean by offense? After all, the United States also believes in the primacy of the offense. Indeed, the only modern state adopting a defensive strategy was France prior to World War II—not a positive advertisement for a defensive approach.

Soviet offensive strategy is above all else methodical. It seeks small bites from the enemy to digest before moving on. This is called "annihilation in detail." Enemy units are first surrounded and then destroyed. The Soviets will only then move on to the next increment of the enemy. The means of surrounding an enemy unit is called the "main blow"—a carefully constructed offensive designed to isolate the target elements of the enemy front lines. Proper calculation of the COF can dictate the place and time for the main blow—assuring a decisive advantage when and where it's needed. The concept of a main blow is not new in Soviet thinking. The Tsarist General Dragomirov specified this approach in 1904—its origins lying in classic Napoleonic warfare as described by Jomini. Soviet encirclement and annihilation of German troops at Stalingrad between November 1942 and February 1943 was an example of this strategy.

Soviet World War II strategy was consistent with Marxist political strategy. It sought to cut apart and isolate enemy coalitions. Each element can then be dealt with piecemeal. Conflict becomes a series of offensive encirclements. Marshal Sokolovskiy's classic 1960s book, *Soviet Military Strategy*,[25] clarifies this concept: "Our strategy adhered to the principle of a progressive destruction of the [enemy] coalition, with the main efforts to be directed each time against the enemy who was most dangerous under the specific conditions and whose destruction would yield the major military and political results on the subsequent course of the war."[26] Soviet strategy in both the Russian Civil War and World War II followed these dicta; it entailed repeated blows—constantly increasing—until the enemy was totally destroyed.

The Soviets have always stressed integrated strategies—rejecting primary reliance on any single weapon or service. Western strategists like Douhet and Fuller, respectively advocates of strategic airpower and tank warfare, were widely read and criticized.[27] For example, the Soviet Union made little use of long-range bomber attacks during World War II.[28] Both during and after that war the Soviets emphasized their integrated strategy, with primacy going to the Red Army—the ultimate instrument of victory. Other forces and forms of warfare support the Red Army by paving the way for the main blow.

In World War II and before, the primary supporting element of the Soviet military was the artillery. Significantly, Peter the Great is touted as the father of Soviet artillery strategy.[29] During World War II airpower increasingly took over the artillery's support role for the Red Army—a sort of long-range artillery. In the words of a World War II Soviet military writer,

"Air superiority is not an end in itself, but for the benefit of the ground troops."[30]

The Soviets have adopted another Clausewitzian principle—the primary objective of war being the annihilation of the enemy army. In this respect the Soviet goal is not the occupation of enemy territory, but the total destruction of enemy forces. Soviet strategists of the 1930s cited Lenin on this point: "Lenin himself believed that the key in the enemy country, that is to say that which guarantees victory, is not the occupation of a part of the hostile country nor the fact of forcing the army of the opponent to abandon his position, but the annihilation, the destruction of the hostile armed forces."[31]

On the eve before the dawn of the nuclear age, the Soviet Union maintained the following military views:

1. The Red Army is the primary military instrument; other military forces play supporting roles.

2. Piecemeal annihilation of enemy forces is the goal, through successive offensive encirclements.

3. The objective is to annihilate enemy military forces.

These ideas persist in today's Soviet strategy, as seen through a nuclear prism.

For almost a decade after World War II, the Soviets publicly belittled nuclear weapons. This approach was not unique to this particular new weapon. As outlined by Henry Kissinger in 1957, Soviet attitudes toward new weapons typically follow three phases:[32]

1. Protestations that new weapons cannot alter basic principles.

2. An about-face to absolute reliance on the new weapons.

3. Integration of the new weapon into an overall strategy.

The first phase lasted until the mid-1950s in the case of nuclear weapons—ending with Stalin's death and Soviet acquisition of their own formidable nuclear capability. The second period lasted until the late 1960s. Since then the Soviets have followed a course which resembles in most respects the US flexible response strategy—integrating nuclear and non-nuclear capabilities.

Stated rejection of the decisiveness of a new weapon, along with a quiet integration of that weapon into the force posture, illustrates Soviet skepticism for single-weapon strategies.[33] The Soviets got the atomic bomb in 1949 and the hydrogen bomb in 1953. But nuclear weapons received little official attention other than strident calls for their complete abolition. Despite this apparent nonchalance, Soviet leaders were terrorized by Western monopolies of nuclear weapons—so much so that they did not inform the Soviet public of Hiroshima until the mid–1950s.[34]

It seems that a rare Soviet strategic debate occurred after Stalin's death. Nothing before or since in Soviet strategy shows such clear evidence of high-level strategic disagreement. The debate had one side seeing the end of the world in nuclear weapons and pressing for a MAD approach. In words that echo Western physicists' dire warnings, some high Soviet officials of the 1950s, such as Chief of the Soviet Council of Ministers G.M. Malenkov (who held a position similar to the White House Chief of Staff) said that a world war would mean "the destruction of world civilization."[35] This school argued for a minimum deterrent—freeing military assets for economic development. On the other side of the debate were those seeking to place the new weapon in the service of greater Soviet military power.

It is probably naive to believe that the 1950s argument could have turned out other than a decision to strengthen Soviet military power. Regardless, the debate was over by 1960 when Khrushchev announced a new military doctrine based on the supremacy of nuclear weapons delivered on ballistic missiles. A new military service—the Strategic Rocket Troops—was formed to manage the new weapon.

The Soviets were not reticent in talking about their strategy during the 1960s. They published a most remarkable book, *Soviet Military Strategy*, in 1962, revising it in 1963 and again in 1968. Nominally attributed to Chief of the Soviet General Staff Marshal V.D. Sokolovskiy, it was a compendium of articles by several senior Soviet authors.[36] This book and others formed the basis of a Soviet Officer's Library to be thoroughly studied and understood by all Soviet officers.

One key factor in Soviet openness during the 1960s was growing confidence in their own technical capability. Soviet Premier Khrushchev's actions and threats to "bury" the United States may not seem credible from a 1990s' perspective. But in the 1960s the Soviets did make major technological break- throughs. They developed the hydrogen bomb as a usable weapon prior to the United States and had the ICBMs to deliver the new weapon considerably before their adversaries. The Soviets launched the first earth-orbiting satellite and put the first man into space. In Marshal Sokolovskiy's words:

> The Soviet Union created the most powerful rockets in the world—the carriers of cosmic objects. The Soviet Union was the first in the world to create the hydrogen bomb and the intercontinental ballistic missile, and also a number of new kinds of rocket armaments which are new in princi- ple.[37]

It was not until the US 1969 manned moon landing that the Soviets became less technologically cocky. It seems that Soviet aggressiveness was motivated in some degree by a perceived technological trend in their favor.

Sokolovskiy's strategy was very much one of nuclear war- fighting. But, despite nuclear weapons' power, it was not a rad- ical departure from traditional Russian and Soviet military approaches. It is significant that Soviet missile forces are called "troops." Sokolovskiy said: "They [nuclear weapons] have enormous destructive capability which, for the first time in his- tory, converts weapons from means of supporting and assuring the combat activities of troops into means of independent fulfill- ment of operational and strategic missions."[38] In short, Soviet strategy was what it had always been, but nuclear-armed rockets assumed the role previously held by divisions, armies, and fronts.

The Soviets recognized the potential of nuclear weapons to change the dynamics, if not the strategy, of war. Sokolovskiy stressed the significance of the opening moves in a nuclear rocket war. Yet strategic targets remained the armed might of the enemy and his means to support it. These targets included the enemy's war economy, command and control, strategic nuclear forces, and other military capabilities.[39]

Even with the Strategic Rocket Troops on top, the Soviets did not retreat from a combined and unified strategy. Right behind the nuclear forces in priority stood the ground forces. Their mission was to "mop up" in order to make the victory complete. Sokolovskiy's words once again were these:

> Final defeat of enemy troops, capture of his territory, the establishment of proper order and peaceful control over all problems after the war can be attained only as a result of combined operation of ground troops.[40]

> It must be taken into account that the most important principle of Soviet military art—victory in war by the combined forces of all services of the armed forces and all means of armed conflict with maximum utilization of the combat capabilities—remains in force at the present time.[41]

The facet of Soviet nuclear strategy which got the most attention in the West—which indeed has become an obsession—is the preemptive strike. The Soviets believe that the West will start a nuclear war, as it was the "West" which started World War II. To avoid their World War II horror, the Soviets are ready to preempt—to get the jump on the West. There is one passage from Sokolovskiy known to every US senator on the Armed Services Committee: "Thus, possibilities exist not to allow a surprise attack by an aggressor: to deliver nuclear strikes on him at the right time."[42] In the United States this preemptive strategy is often confused with a first strike or "bolt from the blue" attack. But the Soviets are clearly talking about a crisis situation of the gravest nature. To the Soviets, preemptive strikes come under the heading of strategic defense—a topic I will discuss later in this chapter.

Since the 1960s, Soviet strategy has evolved slowly. As the number of nuclear weapons and nuclear powers grew—most of whom aim their weapons at the Soviets—the risks of a war in which the Soviets would lose or be gravely damaged also grew. Recent Soviet military writings have been increasingly critical of Sokolovskiy's massive ICBM exchange scenarios.[43] The Soviets have come to see a possibility, and even a necessity, of military victory through non-nuclear means. This realization may well underlie 1980s Soviet enthusiasm for nuclear arms reductions. I believe, though, that arms control has become the "main blow" of Soviet strategy rather than a supporting element as it was in the past.

Other than in the brief flirtation of the 1950s, the Soviets consistently rejected MAD. At the 1967 Glassboro summit Soviet Premier Kosygin called Secretary of Defense McNamara an "immoral capitalist" for espousing it.[44] Sokolovskiy identified MAD targeting of populations as prima facie evidence of Western aggressiveness. Western arms controllers cite the ABM Treaty as evidence of formal Soviet acceptance of MAD. The US ABM Treaty negotiator, Gerard Smith, told Congress during the Treaty ratification hearings that the Treaty represented Soviet adoption of MAD.[45] If the subsequent Soviet offensive buildup and abiding focus on strategic defense does not put a lie to this myth, recent Soviet statements should. During the 1986 Geneva Nuclear and Space Arms Talks, the Soviets specifically pointed to a book by their Deputy Foreign Minister, V. Petrovskiy, which stated: "The Soviet Union opposes maintaining a situation of 'Mutually Assured Destruction' and maintaining peace on that basis."[46]

Despite Soviet rejection of MAD, they accept the idea that prospects of assured destruction—at least for the Western "aggressor"—enhance deterrence. The Soviets do not reject the deterrent effect of MAD, but, rather, they reject is as a basis for strategic thought. MAD is a last resort for them as a deterrent, if all else fails. The only circumstance the Soviets identify MAD as the primary deterrent for is a Western "bolt from the blue"—a possibility even the Soviets take as vanishingly small. Like their Western counterparts, the Soviets have set destruction levels for assured destruction. Characteristically, the Soviet levels—70 percent of US industry and 50 percent of the people destroyed—are larger than Western MAD numbers.[47] Interestingly enough, the Soviets have set this value very near what their current offensive force can do—calculated by the methodology I provided in chapter 1.

Far more important than assured destruction is the Soviet warfighting analysis—the nuclear correlation of forces. During the 1960s the basic scenario and analyses were developed by Major General Anureyev.[48] The analysis starts with precise quantitative measures of opposing sides' reliable and deliverable equivalent megatonnage (EMT) following a preemptive strike by one of them. It measures capability for damage beyond that done against the other's nuclear forces. In short, it measures the relative military power of both. This contrasts with a US approach which concerns itself almost solely with how much damage the United States could do to the Soviet military. The 1960s Soviet COF equations, while modified since then, remain the basis for their strategic calculations.[49] Rather than repeat those complicated equations here, I give a simplified version: ˙

$$COF \ = \ \frac{EMT_{SU} \times PTP \times PS}{EMT_{US} \times PTP \times PS}$$

Where EMT is the total effective megatonnage each side has, PTP is the probability of overcoming the defenses and PS is the probability of non-destruction on the ground in the preemptive strike.

Where do we and the Soviets stand today? That answer is, unfortunately, not encouraging for the United States. Soviet EMT is almost twice US levels (total Soviet megatonnage is almost five times US megatonnage).[50] I've used equivalent megatonnage rather than total megatonnage for the reasons I discussed in chapter 2—EMT is more important in the context of target destruction in a warfighting strategy. I adopt the following values for EMT based on published information and reasonable estimates:

Percent of EMT by Type of Delivery Vehicle

	Soviet (%)	United States (%)
Sub-launched	20	30
ICBMs	70	30
Bombers	10	40

I set overall Soviet active defense effectiveness, including air and missile defenses, conservatively at 20 percent for reasons I discussed in chapter 3. The United States has essentially zero defense. How likely nuclear forces are to be destroyed in a preemptive strike is hotly debated and depends on whether the forces were "generated"—i.e., whether they had any warning to get ready. If generated, they would have been dispersed and ready to go at a moment's notice. For example, missile subs would leave ports, some bombers would go on airborne alert, and others would disperse to remote locations. In my example, I assume no warning and thus "ungenerated" conditions. Recalling from chapter 3 that US Damage Expectancy (DE) is about 0.6 and Soviet DE is about 0.9, I can estimate what percentage of each side's forces would be caught on the ground.

Against the United States, the Soviets could destroy essentially all of our ICBMs on the ground. Those subs in port—roughly one third—would also be gone, and I assume that half of the bombers would escape. About 50 percent of the US forces would survive the preemptive strike, so PS = 0.5.

For the Soviet Union, heavy reliance on ICBMs makes them potentially more vulnerable. Balanced against this is the low US capability—embodied in our low Damage Expectancy—to exploit Soviet vulnerabilities. Increased Soviet emphasis on mobile systems will further reduce this vulnerability. I believe that in the best of circumstances the United States might destroy 40 percent of the Soviet forces. Of course, there are no plans for such a strike, so the calculation is only meaningful because it is how the Soviets figure balances of power. Thus, PS = 0.6 for the USSR.

If I put in these relative numbers, the summary COF equation looks as follows:

$$COF = \frac{2 \times 1.0 \times 0.6}{1 \times 0.8 \times 0.5} = 3.0$$

In short, if we went to war today the Soviet Union would "win" by their calculation—and with a large margin for error. This COF advantage of between 3 and 4 has been confirmed by a number of analyses.[51]

Strategic Defense in Soviet Strategy

In public discussions of the SDI, supporters of the program frequently cite a massive Soviet investment in strategic defense. For example, the US Government released a glossy PR pamphlet in 1985 entitled *Soviet Strategic Defense*.[52] It has long been clear that defenses play a major role in Soviet strategy. They spend at least as much on strategic defenses as they do on strategic offensive forces.[53] A separate military service—the "PVO Strany" or "National Air Defense"—was formed in 1948, third in priority behind the Strategic Rocket Troops and Red Army, but ahead of the Soviet Air Force and Navy.[54]

Soviet interest in strategic defense has led some to propose that they would be receptive to a wholly defensive strategy. Freeman Dyson's eloquent observation that the Soviets should certainly prefer live Russians to dead Americans is one such example.[55] Indeed, the 1986 summit meeting in Reykjavik, Iceland featured a US President earnestly pushing this approach. Both superpowers were to progressively eliminate offensive weapons and then substitute defensive capabilities as the basis of national security. Official US policy expressed this hope: "We must ... negate the destabilizing growth of Soviet offensive forces and ... channel longstanding propensities for defense toward more stabilizing and mutually beneficial ends."[56]

These optimistic hopes of Soviet readiness for a defensive relationship are just that—hopes. The Soviet Union consistently and passionately rejects defensive strategies as certainly as it rejects MAD. Marshal Sokolovskiy wrote of defensive strategies: "Strategic defense and defensive strategy should be decisively rejected as being extremely dangerous to the country."[57] Statements like this, which run throughout Soviet writings, make it clear that the Soviets will accept a defensive strategy only if coerced.

If the Soviet Union rejects defensive strategies, why does it have an abiding interest and investment in this area? The answer lies in the Clausewitzian underpinning to their doctrine. Defenses buy time in order to prepare and launch an offensive and, as such, defenses are an integral part of an offensive strategy. The Soviets emphasize this role even more strongly in the nuclear era. Sokolovskiy believed the lines between strategic offense and defense were becoming increasingly blurred: "Strategic offense and strategic defense as forms of strategic operations under conditions of nuclear rocket war have lost their previous significance."[58]

Soviet insistence on the offensive character of SDI follows directly from the view that defenses must be part of an offensive military strategy. Soviet diatribes against the program feature this argument. Consider one of their 1986 tracts: "The true purpose of the 'strategic defense initiative' is to obtain an opportunity for launching a nuclear attack with impunity, and for continuously harassing the Soviet Union and other countries by means of nuclear blackmail."[59]

During the Russian Civil War and World War II, two types of defensive operations emerged. The first type was the classic Clausewitzian defensive action in order to buy time for an offensive move. The best description of this type of move is Lenin's comment, cited earlier in this chapter, after the Russian "capitulation" to the Germans in the Treaty of Brest-Litovsk, which got them out of World War I: "There are times when we must take one step backward, in order to take two steps forward."[60] The Soviets believed it reasonable then to cede territory in order to buy time. Their choice of a defensive strategy was based on calculations that the COF did not favor an offensive at that time. When it once again became favorable, the Soviets quickly moved to the attack. An interesting testimony to the integral role of defenses in an offensive strategy is the fact that the Soviets initiated an award in 1942 for excellence in retreat—the "Order of Kutuzov"—the only nation in the world to reward that activity.[61]

The second role of defenses in Soviet strategy relates to the concept of the "rear." Far more than the West, the Soviets recognize the need for productive rear areas supplying the vital weapons and men for battle. Strategic defenses have the important job of protecting these rear areas. During World War II Soviet air defenses focused on defending strategic targets against bombers—there was little attention to overall area defense.[62] This point defense mentality persists to this day.

Although the National Air Defense (PVO) was established in 1948, it was not until the mid–1950s that an effective air defense capability was seriously considered.[63] This interest in defense was simultaneous with Soviet adoption of their nuclear-reliant offensive missile strategy. Although the Soviets said little in the 1950s about missile defense possibilities, there can be little doubt that they started work on such defenses at the same time they began developing offensive missiles. By 1961, the

Soviets were ready to publicly announce their missile defense accomplishments. At the 22nd Congress of the Communist Party of the Soviet Union (CPSU) in 1961, Soviet Defense Minister Malinovskiy stated, "The problem of destroying missiles in flight has been solved."[64]

During the 1960s the Soviets pursued three systems with some ABM potential.[65] They deployed the "Griffon" system around Leningrad. This was a forerunner of the Soviet SA-5 air defense system and it may have been "dual mode." This means it could intercept both high-altitude aircraft and ballistic missiles. In the early 1960s the Soviets constructed a line of SA-5 interceptors along ICBM warhead approach corridors in the Northwest USSR. NATO labeled this system "Tallinn" because it originally appeared near the Estonian city of that name. Whether or not these two systems had ABM potential was hotly debated—but they surely represented one Soviet approach to the problem, upgrading air defenses for ABM purposes.

The Soviets did develop and deploy one indisputable ABM in the 1960s—the "Galosh" system around Moscow.[66] In the 1964 Moscow May Day parade, the Galosh interceptor was paraded through the streets. Major construction of Galosh defenses for Moscow began in 1965, continuing through 1967. In 1968 the Soviets stopped work on the Moscow system, having completed only half of what originally looked like a 128-interceptor system. The Galosh was an "exo-atmospheric" nuclear intercept system—it intercepted its target outside the atmosphere, destroying it with a large nuclear warhead.

The Soviets seemed to have had a change of heart on ABMs in 1967. Some experts allege that there was a "debate" over ABMs between those advocating an offensive strategy and those advocating a defensive one. This debate was more likely manufactured for the Western world, which avidly sought, as it still does, evidence of pluralism in Soviet decisionmaking.[67] It is more likely that Defense Secretary McNamara's September 1967 announcement that we were proceeding with our Sentinel ABM system, was the dominant factor in Soviet thinking about ABM.

Prior to 1967 the Soviets sang the praises of defense and defensive strategies. As I have already pointed out, Kosygin blasted McNamara as an immoral capitalist for opposing ABMs at the 1967 Glassboro summit. Perhaps the most remarkable article during this "ABM spring" was one by Major General N. Talenskiy. General Talenskiy had been the editor of the Soviet General Staff classified journal *Military Thought*, and had been instrumental during the 1940s and 1950s in overall Soviet strategy development. His article, "Anti Missile Systems and the Problem of Disarmament," was published in Russian in October 1964. The *Bulletin of the Atomic Scientists* republished it in English in February 1965. General Talenskiy's frequent involvement in Western debates on strategic issues, along with the publication of his article in an arms control enthusiast's magazine, suggests that an element of propaganda was certainly present.[68] Nonetheless, Kosygin's repetition of Talenskiy's arguments at Glassboro suggests that his views came from the top in Moscow.

Talenskiy argued for a defensive strategy in terms similar to those used by President Reagan in the 1980s. In particular, he stressed the possibility that defenses could militarily obsolesce offensive missiles: "I think it is theoretically and technically quite possible to counterbalance the absolute weapons of attack with equally absolute weapons of defense, thereby objectively eliminating war regardless of the desires of resisting governments."[69]

On the role of defenses to enhance deterrence he said: "From the standpoint of strategy, powerful deterrent forces and an effective anti-missile defense system, when taken together, substantially increase the stability of mutual deterrence, for any partial shifts in the qualitative and quantitative balance of these two component elements of mutual deterrence tend to be correspondingly compensated and equalized."

On the superiority of defensive deterrence Talenskiy maintained that: "The creation of an effective anti-missile system enables the state to make its defenses dependent chiefly on its own possibilities, and not only on mutual deterrence, that is the good will of the other side." Finally, on the intentions of those opposing defenses, he concluded: "Only the side which intends to use its means of attack for aggressive purposes can wish to slow down the creation and improvement of anti-missile defense systems.''

After 1967 the Soviets stopped touting defenses in general, and focused on the aggressive nature of US defenses. The fact that this change of heart occurred simultaneously with announcement of a US defensive deployment is not coincidental. The Soviet agreement to enter negotiations on defenses came within weeks of the US decision to deploy the improved Safeguard ABM. Their interests in defenses in the late 1960s were clearly on how to stop US programs—and not to reject defenses for themselves. Soviet activities during the 1969 US ABM debate are interesting and closely parallel their anti-SDI work in the 1980s. They invariably lift their public arguments from the writings of Western critics—who are usually touted as "sober" and "realistic."[70] In the 1960s, the Soviets formulated eight arguments:[71]

1. ABM systems would be too costly.

2. Spending money on defenses would divert US resources from pressing social needs.

3. ABM systems would be ineffective—less than 10 percent effective.

4. ABM systems would exacerbate the arms race—opening new areas for competition.

5. ABM systems are being pushed by profiteers from the US military-industrial complex.

6. ABM systems would make offensive arms control talks more difficult.

7. ABM systems would spur development of new offensive systems.

8. The United States, even if it says it will deploy only a modest defense, would press for a full "heavy" nation-wide defense.

These arguments helped convince the US negotiating team in the ABM talks that they were "educating" the Soviets on the virtues of MAD. The ABM Treaty was signed in 1972, and it stopped US ABM efforts, but did little to slow Soviet work in this area. The Soviets had long since decided that the Galosh was ineffective and had already stopped construction. By agreeing not to build a system they didn't want, the Soviets had halted a potent new US move.

Since 1972, Soviet defense efforts have continued unabated.[72] Once the Soviets solved the technical shortcomings of Galosh in the 1970s, they rebuilt the Moscow system in the early 1980s. The new system was a two-layer system brought up to the full force of 100 interceptors allowed by the ABM Treaty. One type of interceptor is an improved version of the exo-atmospheric Galosh—but now protected by silos; the second type operates inside the atmosphere as an "endo-atmospheric" system. The new Soviet Moscow defenses bear some superficial resemblance to the old US Safeguard. Perhaps the most ominous feature of the new Soviet work is the fact that the endo-atmospheric interceptor has been developed as a mobile capable system—the ABM-X-3. Along the same lines, and following the old Soviet tack of upgrading air defenses for ABM, the SA-10 and SA-12 air defense systems have been developed as dual mode anti-tactical ballistic missile systems and anti-aircraft systems. Thousands of these are being deployed throughout the Soviet Union.

The mobile ABM-X-3 and SA-12 systems take on particular significance in light of Soviet ABM sensor development. The ABM Treaty recognized that radar sensors for ABM systems are the long pole in the ABM tent. For this reason, the Treaty strictly limited ABM radars and missile attack warning radars. A comprehensive long-range radar system could help even the relatively ineffective short-range radars associated with the SA-12 support an effective ABM system. The long-range radar could hand over tracking information, "tipping off" the short-range SA-12 radar that a target was on the way and where to look for it. If the Soviets had such data, US experts believe, the SA-12 and the ABM-X-3, if the Soviets choose to deploy it, could be effective against US strategic warheads—particularly SLBM warheads which have a trajectory not unlike some tactical ballistic missiles.

The Soviets have constructed the long-range radar net necessary to support such a system—its keystone being the

Krasnoyarsk radar in central Siberia, in a location expressly forbidden by the ABM Treaty. Due to its long-lead construction time—ten years or more—the Soviets must have begun this radar about the time they signed the ABM Treaty. This is a significant violation—and one foreseen by the ABM Treaty drafters as a signal of possible ABM breakout precisely because it can support a nationwide defense. These and other facts have led the United States to fear that the Soviet Union is preparing to break out of the ABM Treaty. Worse still, they could do so on short notice and come up with an effective ABM defense.

In addition to their rapidly deployable systems, the Soviets have maintained a vigorous ABM research program. Every element of SDI has a Soviet analogue. However, Soviet efforts, particularly in laser research, have been much larger and in existence much longer than their US counterparts.

Soviet interest in strategic missile defense obviously did not end with the Treaty. On signing it, Soviet Defense Minister Grechko noted that it "did not place any limitations on carrying out research and experimental work toward solving the problem of defense of the country against nuclear attack."[73] Soviet National Air Defense forces remained third in priority, behind the Strategic Rocket Troops and the Army, but ahead of Soviet Air Forces and the Navy. Their share of the Soviet defense budget also remained constant (before and after 1972) at 12-15 percent.[74] As evidence of the continuing importance of missile defense, Marshal of Aviation G.V. Zimin, Chief of the Military Command Academy of the National Air Defense, said in 1976 that it would be necessary to utilize, "the coordinated activity by anti-aircraft, anti-missile, and anti-space defense."[75] Soviet 1980s attacks on the SDI follow closely the late 1960s pattern. They have been particularly active in promoting the virtues of "sober minded" Western critics.

Despite Soviet claims as to the futility of US missile defenses, they are optimistic about their own defenses. They remain confident that the dialectics of a defense for every offense will continue to operate.[76] Note some statements:

1962 Marshal Sokolovskiy—"In the building of the armed forces of the USSR, it is necessary to consider all the trends of development in enemy armed forces in order that there be a countermeasure for each new type of weapon developed by the enemy.''[77]

1964 Major General Talenskiy—''Every decisive new means of attack inevitably leads to the development of a new means of defense.''[78]

1982 Marshal N.V. Ogarkov, Chief of the General Staff—''The experience of past wars convincingly demonstrates that the appearance of new means of attack has always invariably led to the creation of corresponding means of defense.... This applies fully even to the nuclear missile weapons.''[79]

In the context of the US offensive threat, the Soviet Union already has a ''three-layer'' defense. The first ''layer'' is Soviet preemptive strike capability. As I pointed out earlier, it could destroy perhaps 50 percent of US forces before they left the ground. The second defensive layer is Soviet air and missile defense, which I have conservatively estimated to be 20 percent effective. The final Soviet defensive layer is their civil defense. As I described in chapter 1, even simple civil defense can reduce casualties by half. If these three layers are taken together, the Soviet Union has today a better than 80 percent effective defense—compared to an almost zero US defense.

Disarmament: The Soviet ''Main Blow''

We always tell the truth to our friends as well as our enemies. We are in favor of detente, but if anybody thinks that for this reason we shall forget about Marx, Engels, and Lenin, he is mistaken. This will happen when shrimps learn to whistle.... We are for co-existence because there is in the world a capitalist and a socialist system, but we shall always adhere to the building of Socialism ... we don't believe that war is necessary to that end. Peaceful competition will be sufficient.[80]

Nikita Khrushchev
17 September 1955

The most potent Soviet weapon is not military but political. It has a long history: ''The Soviet delegation is convinced that total disarmament ... is the most enduring, the most effective and the most universally accepted security guarantee.''[81]

M.M. Litvinov,
Soviet Foreign Minister
19 March 1928

Peace and complete disarmament have been the basis of Soviet foreign policy since there was a Soviet Union. The first official decree of the Soviet Government was Lenin's "Decree on Peace," 28 October 1917.[82] Soviet diplomats and leaders, starting with Lenin, and including such "peace-loving" leaders as Stalin, down to the current Glasnost-spouting Gorbachev, hammer relentlessly on the need for disarmament. Every Soviet arms control proposal is a step toward complete and total disarmament. These pleas are too frequent and too consistent to be mere propaganda. How do we square this "peace activism" with the Soviet armed forces—the most powerful and massive armed force in the history of mankind?

The answer lies in the unique Soviet blend of Clausewitz and Marxism-Leninism. There are three basic principles:

1. Marx and Lenin teach that all conflicts grow out of class struggle. Hence, the adoption of the Clausewitzian dictum that war is politics by other, violent means. Further, this class struggle, or "war," is one Socialism is destined to win.

2. Marxism-Leninism arms its adherents with "scientific" tools with which to pursue their political goals. In conflict this translates into scientific calculation of the COF. But this same "scientific" approach is even more successful in economic and political competition.

3. Uncertainty ruins this method. Clausewitz maintains that the greatest uncertainty is "friction," the unpredictability of events during combat. War is to be avoided by Marxists. During war the "scientific" method is most unreliable because there is the most uncertainty.

From these principles it follows that the Soviets believe they are locked into a historical conflict—one they are destined to win. Their "scientific" method gives them a decisive advantage, they believe. Yet, uncertainty—the throw of the dice in war—could ruin everything. The best bet for Soviet victory is thus a disarmed world.

The danger of uncertainty permeates Soviet military writings.[83] In the 1960s, as represented in Sokolovskiy's writings and the quantitative COF equations of Anureyev, the Soviets toyed with the idea that nuclear war might be handled in a quantitative, predictable manner. It now appears that this view has fallen aside. The Soviets seem to have decided that nuclear war poses too many risks to fit into Marxist philosophy. Sokolovskiy said that nuclear weapons do not change the basic Clausewitzian dictum: "It is well known that the essence of war as a continuation of politics does not change with changing technologies and armament."[84] More recent writings, however, take a much different tack: "It is precisely in this [nuclear-space] sense that it is correct to consider that Clausewitz's formula is obsolete; according to which 'war is nothing but the continuation of state policy by other means.'"[85]

The abandonment of nuclear war as an instrument of policy has led to increasingly insistent demands for nuclear disarmament. This by no means indicates Soviet abandonment of their long-term historical goals. The Soviets are quite willing to compete in other areas of military and political power. My analysis in the introduction shows that space will soon be more important than nuclear weapons. The Soviets have every intent to compete in this area, as I discuss at the end of this chapter. A few sentences after V. Petrovskiy's rejection of Clausewitz in nuclear war, above, he reiterated that the basic concept, "War is politics," remains valid in "the social and philosophical context of this definition."[86] To understand this, we must consider what the Soviets mean by "peaceful coexistence."

Khrushchev made it clear in the late 1950s that peaceful coexistence meant that the Soviets would beat the West by peaceful means. Their recent views, as stated by Petrovskiy in 1985, are the same: "For the Socialist countries, peaceful coexistence—or as V.I. Lenin used to say, 'living together peacefully'—with the bourgeois states is a strategic task of foreign policy, because solving this problem gives the best external conditions for socialist and communist upbuilding."[87]

These latest writings do not exclude military action from peaceful coexistence: "Of course, peaceful coexistence, which is the basis for relationships between states with a different situation, is by no means equivalent to recognizing the social status quo and denying peoples the right to wage a campaign for their social and national liberation.''[88]

As for who needs ''liberation'' the Soviets said that: ''NATO has in its arsenal an entire system of measures aimed at the 'collective' suppression of people in the NATO nations, who would otherwise have decided to break with capitalism and make sweeping social and economic changes.''[89]

One point to keep in mind when listening to Soviet ideas is the two linked concepts—*peace* and *security*. The former is the absence of war—the latter is the absence of things that cause war. The Soviets insist on having both. It is wise to keep in mind that the Soviets have not abandoned the view that class struggle causes war. We cannot have security, in their opinion, until the class struggle is ended.[90]

What is the basic weapon in the Soviet ''peaceful coexistence'' arsenal? In my opinion it is not the Soviet armed forces—although they certainly support Soviet goals—but it is arms control. Invariably, the Soviets praise all Western acquiescence to arms control.[91]

If arms control is their objective, what then is the role of their nuclear forces? The Soviets have also made this clear. They consider it their greatest accomplishment to have achieved the COF advantage over the West—and they intend to use this advantage. The 1980 Plenum of the CPSU made this very clear:[92]

> The strategic military balance of power which has been attained between the world of socialism and the world of capitalism is a victory of historic scope and deep principle. It serves as a factor for restraining the aggressive aspirations of imperialism which corresponds to the basic interests of all peoples.
>
> By depriving the United States of the capability of blackmailing the Soviet Union and other countries with a nuclear threat, strategic military balance of power makes possible a consolidation of the foundations of peaceful coexistence.

In short, the Soviets intend to use their advantage to force disarmament on their terms—which means they can continue their historic struggle undeterred by the threat of an unpredictable war.

Soviet Views on the Military Use of Space

> Space supremacy is the aim of the next decade. The country that controls space can control the Earth.
> Attributed to President Kennedy in *Soviet Military Strategy*, 1st edition, V.D. Sokolovskiy, 1962[93]

This incorrectly quoted thought shows early and abiding Soviet fear of US space activities. Earlier Soviet musings regarded space as a new area for competition—and one in which the Soviets were confident that they would prevail. Soviet space successes—Sputnik and the first manned space flight—certainly gave them cause for optimism. By the late 1960s, US space successes showed that the trend in space was not moving in favor of the Soviets. As they have done so often this century, they turned to their most reliable weapon to redress the problem— arms control.

With the aid of arms controllers in the West, the Soviets pressed for and got the 1967 Outer Space Treaty.[94] The Treaty bans military use of heavenly bodies and prohibits nuclear weapons and "other" weapons of mass destruction from space. Significantly, the Treaty exempted ballistic missile warheads, which, after all, fly through space, from the class of space weapons. It's clear that the Soviets wanted to exempt the one class of space weapon for which the COF was moving in their favor.

The Soviet Union continues to press for limitations and bans on weapons in space. Since 1967 Soviet military literature has progressively dropped discussion of Soviet military space goals. The usual dodge is to discuss military space possibilities, which they clearly don't want their military people to ignore, under the guise of studying "Western" military ideas. For example, Sokolovskiy's third edition of *Military Strategy* relegated all space discussions to the chapter on Western strategies. The trend in this direction accelerated in the 1980s. Entries in the latest *Soviet Military Dictionary* omit many previously acknowledged military uses of space and transfer those that remain to the category of ''foreign'' programs.[95] In truth, Soviet military activities completely dominate their space effort, and are a vital part of their offensive force posture. For example, Soviet space activities come under the offensive force—the Strategic Rocket Troops.[96] Soviet public denial of such activities often gets ridiculous.[97]

The 1980s saw an increasingly frantic Soviet obsession with US military space programs. In 1979 the Soviets participated in the ASAT talks—which broke down in part over Soviet insistence that the US Space Shuttle was a military weapon. When it became operational in 1981, Soviet diplomatic efforts intensified. In the early 1980s they pushed repeatedly for arms control treaties banning all weapons in space. The SDI program has driven them to new heights of frenzy. Every book or article published against the SDI by the Soviets stresses the space-based portion of the program. I note that General Secretary Gorbachev's top objective at the 1986 Reykjavik summit was to confine the space-based defense work to laboratories—he proposed no such restrictions on ground-based technologies.[98]

Why do the Soviets fear space? The Soviets, I feel, now equate space weapons with nuclear weapons.[99] As I showed in the introduction, the Soviets are well justified in their fear. As I also pointed out (in chapter 1,) it is not the fear of having their cities ''lasered'' that worries them. Soviet propagandists have, however, given away their true concerns. In the words of the Committee of Soviet Scientists for Peace Against the Nuclear Threat in *Space-Strike Arms and International Security,* published just before the November 1985 Geneva summit:

> It is worth mentioning that space strike weapons which are being developed in the USA appear to be intended not only for knocking out the other side's satellites and strategic missiles after the launch but also as pre-emptive weapons to be used against ground targets, for performing the first strike. Accurate and powerful enough to destroy strategic ballistic missiles in flight, space-based weapons can also be used to hit other types of strategic weapons, e.g. planes on airfields before they take off. Besides it has been reported in the American press that space-based strike

weapons could also hit other ground and sea targets, including command posts, communications and control networks, large floating targets and key economic facilities (oil and gas refineries, chemical plants, power stations, etc.).[100]

In actual fact, I could find no press reports which mentioned these military uses against the Soviet Army and its rear areas—US discussion in this period centered only on space weapons with mass destruction potential. Significantly, the conventional military use of space is the only item discussed in Soviet anti-SDI propaganda which does *not* come from United States SDI critics' writings.

A cursory glance at Soviet long-term strategy shows why space weapons are so threatening. As they move away from nuclear strategies, Soviet ground forces retake center stage. As I showed earlier, the Red Army has always been the centerpiece of their strategy. Even in the 1960s—the heyday of Soviet nuclear enthusiasm—its Army maintained a priority only just behind the Strategic Rocket Troops.

Western space capabilities threaten to overturn correlation of forces advantages in both pillars of Soviet strength. Strategic defenses will negate and make obsolete the military significance of the Strategic Rocket Troops. But more importantly, the space "spinoffs" of the Strategic Defense Initiative will provide a potent and decisive tool against the Soviet Army.

Space capabilities could give the United States a potent hand in the next few poker games with the Soviets. Space is the winning card, not just a bargaining chip. The Soviets hope to use politics and arms control to slow or halt US space efforts. Meanwhile, the basic enabling technology—the ability to place lots of mass into orbit—is being rapidly advanced by the Soviets. Under the guise of peaceful space cooperation, the Soviet Union may well achieve a decisive advantage in the parameters which matter most in the correlation of forces analyses of the decades ahead. We ignore these facts and trends to our great peril.

CONCLUSION: US STRATEGIC DEFENSE

A serious challenge faces the United States. We are confronted by a growing power imbalance which many view as unacceptable. Our people seem increasingly less willing to bear the burden of countering foreign military and political threats. Although the circumstances were far different, the final decades of the Roman empire provide some interesting food for thought. I won't speculate on what caused the fall of the Roman empire, but military problems no doubt contributed.[1] Many view US national security as being in serious disarray. Some counsel emphasis on technological fixes,[2] as did an anonymous Roman in the 4th century AD:

> Above all it must be recognized that wild nations are pressing upon the Roman Empire and howling round about it everywhere, and treacherous barbarians, covered by natural positions, are assailing every frontier ... Nations of this kind, then, which are protected by such defenses or by city- and fortress-walls, must be attacked by a variety of new military machines. But in case any difficulty should arise in constructing these types of weapons I have attached to my dialogue a very accurate coloured picture of the hurling engines, so that the task of imitating them may be easy.[3]

Others advocate renewed emphasis on basic military skills,[4] as did a noted Roman general of the same era:

> Victory in war does not depend entirely upon numbers or mere courage; only skill and discipline will ensure it. We find that the Romans owed the conquest of the world to no other cause than continual military training, exact observance of discipline in their camps and unwearied cultivation of the other arts of war.[5]

Advocates of strategic defense often fall into the first category. It is my position, and the subject of this chapter, that these issues, technological or military, cannot and must not be separated from strategy.

Evolving US Strategic Defense Alternatives

In previous chapters I outlined the three basic strategic approaches. In the 1990s, advocates of each will propose strategic deployments. Proponents of specific deployments may or may not have a clear strategic vision. The public debates on each will almost entirely ignore strategy. In this context, I believe debate will focus on three hardware systems—one supporting MAD, one supporting nuclear warfighting, and one supporting non-nuclear, strategic defense-based deterrence.

MAD advocates propose a small, single-warhead mobile missile called "Midgetman." The early 1980s strategic study by the bipartisan Scowcroft Commission advocated Midgetman as a compromise between those who saw the need for new offensive forces to offset Soviet correlation of forces (COF) advantages and those who wanted to move toward a more survivable MAD deterrent.[6] By 1986 Midgetman's cost, near $100 million per warhead, caused the nuclear warfighters to lose interest in Midgetman and to oppose it.[7] They favored more cost-effective multiple warhead systems. If anyone doubts that Midgetman is a MAD system, consider the fact that it has been, cautiously, endorsed by the Union of Concerned Scientists—the only new nuclear weapon to be so blessed.[8] By simple multiplication it would require about $100 billion over the next decade to reach the 1000-warhead level required for MAD. Of course, the Soviets would have to agree to dismantling their dual-purpose air defenses. These defenses are already good enough to threaten the penetrability of a single-warhead system such as Midgetman.[9]

The nuclear warfighters prefer new hard-target kill systems—the Trident D-5 submarine and a mobile M-X ICBM. As I discussed in chapter 2, the United States would need about 2,500 additional warheads to redress the current Soviet COF advantages.[10] The nuclear warfighters could fix their problem for about $75 billion—a cost roughly comparable to the MAD alternative. Of course, the new US offensive systems must be able to survive Soviet preemption and penetrate Soviet defenses if they are to be effective. Soviet defenses worry warfighters.

They fear that a near-term move to deploy strategic defenses would trigger a massive Soviet defensive deployment, and they assume the Soviets could deploy defenses sooner than the United States. The end result would be less US warfighting deterrence. Thus, warfighters take a go-slow attitude on SDI and defensive deployments.[11]

Those favoring strategic approaches not relying on strategic defenses have a convenient excuse, claiming that effective defenses won't be possible for decades. (MAD advocates say many decades, warfighting advocates say a few decades.[12]) These strategists find it convenient to advocate a vigorous *long-term* research program on defenses in the hopes that the whole idea will go away. This is a variant on the 1950s strategy used by defense critics to delay deploying Nike Zeus (see chapter 3). Fortunately, effective defenses are not decades away. By 1986, the SDI program had advanced to the point where the United States could begin deploying defenses in the early 1990s and have them firmly in place by the mid-1990s.[13] The initial defense increments would cost between $50 billion and $100 billion. We can, therefore, discuss now an alternate 1990s strategy based on strategic defenses. The cost and schedule for developing such defenses are comparable to the alternatives.

In the remainder of this chapter I will outline the type of defenses we can have and how they might evolve to support a defensive strategy. In order to meet the policy requirements I outlined, these must have certain technical characteristics. Those translate into whether the defenses are survivable, effective, and cost-effective at the margin. As I discussed in the Introduction, the technical reality of these defenses and the political will to proceed with them could persuade the Soviets to accept the proposed US defensive strategy despite their long-standing antipathy to such defenses. This could happen before any defenses are actually deployed, or at any time in the deployment evolution. The Soviets may well find a cooperative transition to a defense-reliant relationship the least of several evils.

To show how we might move toward a defense-reliant posture, I consider two-and-a-half cycles of offense-defense reactions (which some might call an arms race.) The first cycle would begin when the United States unilaterally deploys a defensive system and end when the Soviet Union responds with an offensive counter.

Suppose the United States develops a defensive system in the mid-1990s. This defense, which I will designate System A, must meet two criteria:

1. It must be good enough to remove the current Soviet correlation of forces advantage—that is, it must deny their current war plan.

2. It must provide a significant decrease in damage to the United States, whose people will be little interested in an initial defense which does not significantly reduce their vulnerability—regardless of its strategic implications. I estimate that a defense which can stop two-thirds of the Soviet arsenal would be accepted as a useful first step.

Against our initial System A, the Soviets would consider five possible responses:

1. Accept a US-proposed, cooperative transition to a defense-dominant world.

2. Recover previous Soviet COF advantage through their own defensive deployments.

3. Recover their previous COF advantage through offensive proliferation.

4. Ignore the near-term System A disadvantage and concentrate on long-term responses to recover their offensive advantage—that is, new offensive system types.

5. Concentrate on defensive suppression measures to negate US defenses when required.

Of course, the Soviets could try a combination of approaches. Fiscal limitations, however, would force them to emphasize one over the others. For the purposes of this analysis, I will address each response separately. Responses one and two would represent US success. If the Soviets chose to ''race'' in building their defenses, the end result would be the defense-dominant world the United States seeks.

Against Soviet response three, offensive proliferation, the United States must be ready to deploy an upgraded defense—

which I will call System B. This upgrade must, at a minimum, maintain the unfavorable Soviet COF which System A caused. System B must be able to do this against an all-out Soviet offensive proliferation.

If the Soviets choose response four, developing "responsive" new offensive systems, the United States must have a long-term option to negate these new types of offensive systems. I call such an advanced defensive system C.

Of course the Soviets might try to suppress the defenses by attacking them. To be "survivable" each defensive system, A, B, and C, must be able to maintain its effectiveness despite determined attacks against it.

Figure 11 is my estimated timeline for each system's deployment and Soviet countermeasures against it. These defensive systems must meet the following quantitative stability requirements:

1. System A must remove the current Soviet COF advantage, and it must remove that advantage at roughly the same cost as proposed US offensive deployments—alternatives to a defensive approach.

2. System B must be "cost-effective at the margin." In other words it must preserve or enhance the COF equalization which System A bought, and it must do this at less cost to the United States than the Soviet offensive counters to it.

3. System C must be similarly cost-effective at the margin against the Soviet offensive response to System B.

4. All three must be survivable, and it must cost less to maintain their effectiveness than to degrade them with defense suppression attacks. I will consider three forms of defense suppression:

—Soviet attempts to deny system deployment.

—Soviet attrition of systems after they have been deployed.

—Soviet preparations to "blow a hole" in the defense as part of a preemptive strike.

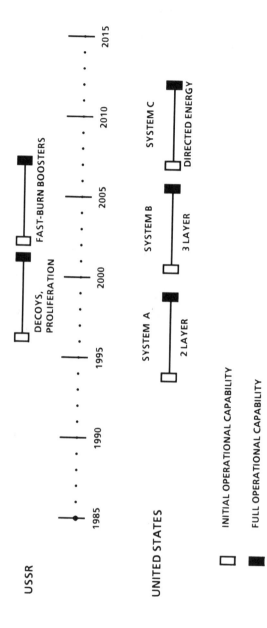

Figure 11. Timeline for Deployment of Proposed US Strategic Defensive Systems and Soviet Responses.

Three Defensive Systems

Many people are confused about different types of missile defense. I don't think the average decisionmaker, let alone interested members of the public, appreciates the subtle differences between "post-boost phase" defenses and "interactively discriminated midcourse" defenses. The missile defense terminology of the 1960s lies at the root of the problem. At that time we categorized defensive systems by the portion of an ICBM's flight where the defensive system operated. In the 1960s ICBMs had three distinct phases.

During the first or "boost" phase the ICBM's rocket engines burned for a few minutes to thrust the single warhead up out of the atmosphere into space and on its way toward its target. Once in space the rocket engine fell away and the warhead proceeded on a "ballistic" arc hundreds of kilometers up and thousands of kilometers long. This "midcourse" phase lasted about 30 minutes for an ICBM. In the final minute of flight the nuclear warhead "reentry vehicle" or "RV" reentered the atmosphere over its target in what is called "terminal" phase.

Offensive nuclear missiles have evolved since the 1960s— rendering this defensive terminology obsolete. Partly as a way to overwhelm the old-style defenses, both the United States and the Soviet Union developed and deployed "Multiple Independently Targetable Reentry Vehicles" (MIRVs). On top of a MIRVed ICBM sits a device carrying three or more warheads. This device is called a "post-boost vehicle" or sometimes just a "bus." The bus has a small rocket engine which fires repeatedly once it gets into space to send each warhead toward a different target. The Soviet SS-18, largest ICBM in their 1990s inventory, can carry 10 or more warheads, each capable of reaching a different target. Figure 12 illustrates the phases of 1990s ballistic missiles of different ranges.

Another possible development would be a "depressed trajectory" missile. If the missile and warhead can stay low enough there is a better chance of slipping under the defender's radar coverage and surprising his defense. To do this the ICBM or submarine-launched ballistic missile (SLBM) is fired at a

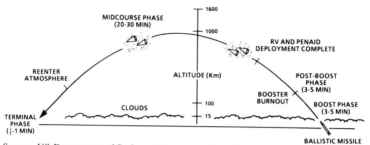

Source: US Department of Defense, Strategic Defense Initiative Organization.

Figure 12. Defensive Intercept Phases. Depicted here are ballistic missile flight phases for a "heavy" Soviet ICBM like the SS-18. The length of phases, altitude of flight, and other features could change considerably in new missile systems designed to be "responsive" to defensive systems.

lower angle so that it stays inside the atmosphere longer and spends less time in space where the radar can see it. This type of countermeasure would be most useful in situations where the defender is relying solely on interception in space.

A third approach for confounding defenses is to give the warhead the ability to maneuver after it has entered the atmosphere in terminal phase. A Maneuvering RV or MaRV can evade certain kinds of defensive systems.

For these reasons I prefer to separate defensive systems into three types divided, not according to the phases of the offensive missile's flight, but according to how the defensive system works and where it's based. My three distinct types of defensive systems are: *Point*, *Sovereign Area*, and *Global*. These systems may overlap in coverage, and may operate during more than one phase of an attacking missile's flight.

To understand how each type of missile defense works, consider US naval defenses in the nineteenth century. We had *Point Defenses* based on shore near our vital harbors in the form of shore batteries. These point defenses defended only a single target and were based near that target. We also had *Sovereign Area Defenses* in our 19th-century Coast Guard consisting of short-range ships—each capable of defending a large part, if not all, of one seaboard. These sovereign area defenses were based in our own territory, but could defend many targets. Finally, our

19th-century blue water navy provided us a *Global Defense*, able to defend the United States or its allies at any place on the globe from attack originating at any other place, provided we had enough notice to concentrate our ships for warding off the attack.

In ballistic missile defense, Point Defenses generally work only in the missile's terminal phase. Sovereign area missile defenses can also operate in terminal phase, but can in addition work during much of the midcourse phase, depending on how soon the sensor system picks up and tracks attacking warheads. In a missile defense system, the global defenses have part, if not all, of their elements based in space. From space they can defend both in boost phase and in midcourse.

The actual hardware in a missile defense system has three parts: sensors, weapons, and battle management. The sensors are the eyes of the system, detecting, identifying and tracking the missile or warhead targets. The battle management part is the brain, using computers to decide which weapon to assign to which target and to keep abreast of the overall engagement. The defensive weapons are the "fists," which do the job of stopping the attacking missiles and warheads.

During the 1960s the United States and Soviet Union both developed missile defense systems. As I described, we deployed our Safeguard missile defense system in the early 1970s at Grand Forks, North Dakota. The Soviet Union deployed their Galosh system in the mid-1960s around Moscow. Safeguard used two different defense systems: Sprint and Spartan. Sprint was a short-range point defense, and it used a small, fast missile as a last-ditch defense just before the attacking warhead hit its target. Spartan had a large missile which flew deep into space to intercept attacking warheads hundreds of kilometers from their targets. Both missiles carried a nuclear warhead and both relied on radars and sophisticated battle management computers.

The 1972 ABM Treaty limited both sides to 100 missile interceptors—the United States chose a mix of Sprint and Spartan missiles in North Dakota. We had barely completed our allowed systems in the mid-1970s when we decided to dismantle them. However, the Soviet Union deployed its Moscow Galosh system and is the process of upgrading it.[14]

The Soviets were deploying, in the late 1980s, a nation-wide "air" defense weapon, the SA-12B, which has the capability to perform tactical ballistic missile intercepts. Many experts believe that "tactical" could extend all the way up to our SLBMs and some ICBMs. One way to make such a system effective against many strategic missiles is to provide it data from long-range early warning radars. The ABM Treaty framers were aware of this potential problem and placed limitations on where and how such long-range radars could be constructed. The Soviet Union violated this provision by constructing a long-range radar at Krasnoyarsk, Siberia. The Soviets have thus used the Krasnoyarsk and other Treaty violations and loopholes to give themselves what many believe to be a formidable point defense system.[15]

Defense System A

My initial system has two defensive layers—one layer a sovereign area defense and the other a global defense. I reject point defenses as part of a defense-reliant deterrent architecture for several reasons. First, once the location and number of interceptors are known, the Soviets can easily calculate how to overwhelm them. They need only target one more warhead than the point defense has interceptors. Second, in order to build an effective point defense to confound Soviet war plans, we must know which targets are most important to those plans. There has been a tendency, as I described in previous chapters, to mirror image US strategy and place strategic missiles at the top of the list. As I discussed earlier, offensive nuclear missiles are no doubt high on Soviet target lists, but other targets also figure prominently. Once we emplace point defenses to protect what *we* think matters to the Soviets, we give away our knowledge of their plans. Armed with this information, it would be easy for the Soviets to modify those plans to attack what we haven't defended. With reliance on global and sovereign area defenses, we needn't know the details of Soviet targeting—just a general idea of their success criteria. Their COF equation is just such a parameter.

Third, there are potent political reasons for rejecting point defenses. Soviet targets are probably not cities per se,[16] but this fact is moot in the minds of the American people. Point defenses designed to protect what the Soviets target, military forces, will not defend people, while area defenses and global defenses protect everything. The only way for point defenses to protect people is to base them in cities. This day-to-day reminder of nuclear war is unacceptable to the American people, as we saw with the riots over the 1960s Sentinel deployment in cities.

I will not provide detailed technical descriptions of the systems and technologies I propose. Such data has been widely disseminated by the Department of Defense.[17] Instead I will give a general outline of a defense system.

The 1970s Spartan, which operated outside the atmosphere ("exoatmospherically"), was a sovereign area defense relying on the large phased-array radar sensor at Grand Forks, North Dakota. This radar still operates and could support a limited area defense. The US early warning system has other parts in the form of modern space-based and ground-based sensors. These sensors could help a central missile-defense radar by providing warhead tracks early in the defensive battle. The earlier the battle manager has this data, the sooner it can commit interceptors. The earlier we commit the interceptors, the larger the area which a single defensive site can defend.

Sensors carried on aircraft can do the sovereign area defense job better than ground-based radars. Airborne sensors have two advantages. First, the mobile aircraft are difficult, if not impossible, for the Soviets to find and destroy. Since the aircraft remain deep in sovereign territory, they are well protected. The large, fixed Safeguard radars were much easier to target and were that system's Achilles' heel. Second, high-altitude sensors have a large sensor range. A single aircraft could cover an area several thousand kilometers across—three to five could defend all of North America. Airborne missile defense sensors would detect and track warheads much as the Airborne Warning and Control System (AWACS) planes direct an air defense battle. The AWACS planes carry radar, but missile-defense planes would use infrared sensors to detect the heat of the incoming warheads. Infrared "television" would pick out the attacking warheads against the "cold"—close to absolute zero—background of deep space. Small lasers carried on the same planes would measure the distance to and speed of the targets. These Airborne Optical Systems (AOS) would send this information to the interceptor missiles—guiding each missile to a target the battle manager had picked out for it. The US Army's Airborne Optical Adjunct Experiment tested some of the technology needed for an AOS in the late 1980s.

The Safeguard defense system, with both Spartan and point defense Sprint missiles, had a sophisticated computer-based battle management system. It also used several million lines of computer code or "software." Some of the code for a sovereign area defense can be resurrected and all of it could be rewritten quickly. The US Army operates a computer center in Huntsville, Alabama where new battle management methods have been constantly developed and upgraded since the early 1970s.

On 10 June 1984, in the Homing Overlay Experiment, a non-nuclear US Army interceptor missile lifted off from the Kwajalein Missile Test Range in the Pacific and sped out into space. A few minutes later, more than 200 kilometers up in space and hundreds of kilometers down range, the interceptor opened its infrared eye and saw the heat of a mock warhead which had been fired several tens of minutes earlier from the Vandenberg Air Force Base in California—thousands of kilometers away. On-board computers directed the interceptor to fire its small rocket and maneuver into the path of the oncoming warhead. The interceptor made a direct hit with the warhead, pulverizing both itself and its target. The SDI program contains a follow up to this experiment—a Ground-Based Interceptor (GBI) designed to intercept its target outside the atmosphere or "exo"-atmospherically. These GBI missiles have been estimated by their developers to weigh about one-thousand kilograms and cost approximately $3 million each—including costs of their ground support equipment and ten years' maintenance.[18] The interceptors would be small enough to be carried on mobile launchers. As with the AOS, these small mobile systems are difficult for the Soviets to find and destroy.

The United States first considered global defenses in 1958 when we began work on a "Ballistic Missile Boost Intercepts" or "BAMBI" system.[19] The idea was good, but the technology was lacking to make BAMBI affordable. By the 1980s technology had caught up with that concept. An SDI experiment team launched two small satellites into orbit atop a Delta rocket on 5 September 1986. Each satellite had its own infrared or radar sensor which collected data as the other satellite maneuvered with its rocket engine. This data will be used to design the best sensor configuration for a space-based missile defense. In a final success, one of the 5 September 1986 satellites homed in and collided with the other satellite that was maneuvering at the time.

The United States could use an improved version of our current early warning satellites as an initial global defense sensor. These early warning satellites are deep in space (geosynchronous orbits) and can see the intense heat of an ICBM or other missile launch with on-board infrared sensors. An upgraded missile defense sensor—the Boost Surveillance and Tracking System or BSTS—could spot boosters within seconds of their launch and transmit this data to the global defense battle management system.

Strategic defense critics have overworked one theme. They claim that reliable software for a missile defense battle management system is impossible. During the 1960s ABM debate several distinguished software experts "proved" that it would be impossible to build the necessary software for Safeguard.[20] Other software experts refuted them—perhaps most effectively by building and deploying a reliable Safeguard software system.[21] Nonetheless, SDI critics have resurrected this old argument in the 1980s—replete with "proofs" of infeasibility by distinguished software experts.[22] Not to be outdone, the Soviets have asserted that a centrally controlled global defense would require 10 billion lines of code and concluded that "such a system can hardly be written."[23]

In 1983, the Defensive Technologies Study Team, or "Fletcher" study, examined the battle management problem for a global defense system.[24] They concluded that a central program of about 10 million (not billion!) lines of computer code would do the trick. Although this is somewhat larger than current military software systems, it is within the state of the art. The Bell Telephone System contains about 50 million lines of code—although it has been written and upgraded over a 20-year period.[25] Like the Bell System, global defense software does not require absolute perfection. Software failures are statistically predictable and can be handled as a design parameter—much as engineers compensate for possible hardware failures by redundancy, alternate paths and system checking. Finally, there are new automated software development and checkout approaches based on technologies such as the misnamed "artificial intelligence."[26]

In 1985 the nation's best software engineers carefully examined the global defense software problem. They agreed that battle management for such systems was feasible and within current US technical capabilities.[27] The reason for their optimism had nothing to do with new technology, but with an adaptation of millennia-old military principles. Military commanders do not rely on 100 percent central control; neither do they allow complete decentralized decisionmaking. Consider General Eisenhower's management of the 1944 D-Day invasion of Normandy. The general did not have a field telephone to every soldier; neither did he let everyone "do his own thing." Instead, he established "hierarchical" control—issuing general instructions to his immediate subordinate commanders, who in turn expanded on the instructions by filling in details. They then transmitted them down to lower levels of command.

A global missile defense would operate similarly. Command and control could be distributed, hierarchically, through the levels of the defensive system. At the top, we would have a redundant, man-in-the-loop central control to set overall requirements. Lower level battle management, perhaps on board the sensor satellites, could divide the defensive engagement into geographic sectors on the globe. Local battle managers, who could be co-located with weapons satellites, could direct the details of the battle in each sector. (This approach can be fully tested at each separate level.) For example, mid-level control can be fully exercised without firing any weapons. If we lose one or more of the elements at any level, that would not bring down the entire system the way that losing central control in a centrally managed system might. Finally, software requirements at any level are relatively modest—a few million lines of code or less, comparable to current strategic military software systems.[28]

Hierarchical battle management systems can be built today. The successful 5 September 1986 space experiment used a battle management system with over one million lines of new code— and the program worked as specified the first time it was tried. The SDI program includes a National Test Bed in Colorado Springs, Colorado for developing and testing hierarchical battle management systems for global missile defenses.

The 5 September 1986 experiment also proved that there are no show-stopping technical obstacles against the initial global defense weapons system. The experiment showed how to build a space-based "kinetic" interceptor. These space-based interceptors, or SBIs, destroy their targets by running into them, that is with kinetic energy. To be effective the SBIs must be small and affordable. Moreover, they must be able to pick out the booster target itself from the much larger signal generated by the booster rocket exhaust or plume. If the interceptor can't identify the actual booster from its plume, it could well miss the target. Each interceptor could weigh as little as 100 kilograms and reside, along with eight or ten of its fellows, on a small sat-ellite carrier. Upon receiving notice of a hostile launch, the interceptors would shoot out of their carrier satellites with instructions on where to look for the targets. Each interceptor would fire its own small rocket motors to home onto and crash into the enemy boosters.

System A's primary objective is to redress the current Soviet COF advantage. From the data I discussed in chapter 3, a defensive system able to stop about two-thirds (66 percent) of the Soviet offensive arsenal would accomplish this objective. This goal allows me to estimate the size of an initial deployment.

The global defense layer has high "leverage." Because a single shot can kill a booster with ten or more warheads, and perhaps many more decoys, this defensive layer has the highest priority. If the global layer could stop 40 percent of a massive Soviet strike, and the sovereign area defense layer stop 40 per-cent of the attackers which got through the global layer, that would meet my overall effectiveness goal for System A. For the purpose of this analysis, I assume that the Soviet strategic attack arsenal could grow to 15,000 warheads by the mid-1990s from its mid-1980s level of about 10,000 nuclear warheads.[29] The Soviet warheads might be carried on 2,000 ICBMs. These levels exceed the SALT limits on Soviet launchers, but it is fair to assume that the Soviets might disregard these limits if they saw it in their national interest to do so. Therefore, the global defense must be able to stop approximately 800 missiles. If I assume that the bulk of the Soviet arsenal will remain on land-based ICBMs as it is today, these 800 missiles must be stopped over the Soviet land mass. I further tilt the analysis in favor of the offense by assuming the Soviets would fire their entire arsenal in a single strike. Their strategy would actually entail several attacking waves of missiles. For reasons I discuss below, attacks spread over time would be easier for the defense to handle.

Massive simultaneous launches are most difficult for a global defense due to the "absentee" problem. Since global defenses orbit elsewhere over the globe, only 15 percent of the constellation would be over the Soviet Union at any given time. Of course, the absentee weapons would be available to stop SLBMs and intermediate-range missiles fired outside the Soviet Union. If the Soviets failed to fire their entire arsenal in less than 10 minutes, new defensive weapons would orbit into position to replace those which were used. In order to threaten 800 Soviet boosters in a single massive Soviet launch of 2,000 boosters, I need 6,000 interceptors in orbit—assuming each has a 90 percent chance of hitting its target. If each carrier satellite carries 10 SBKKV interceptors, this means I need 600 carrier satellites in orbit.

If the above global defense layer did its job, 9,000 Soviet warheads would get through. To meet my requirements, the sovereign area defense must stop 40 percent of these, or 3,600 warheads. Again I assume a 90 percent success rate for each interceptor fired. So I would need 4,000 GBI interceptors based in the United States, along with associated sensors and battle management.

Cost estimates are always tough—DOD officials are constantly reminded of $7,000 coffee pots and $600 hammers. Nonetheless, I can make reasonable cost estimates based on existing defense systems. Table 4 (page 184) lists the elements of System A and the numbers of each element needed. Costs are dominated by the most numerous element—the weapons. In each case I have made my estimates based on existing military systems of similar size and complexity. My estimates are consistent with published external and US Government cost estimates, including some by SDI critics.[30]

To illustrate my costing methodology, consider the SBI weapons. US experience has shown that the key and almost only cost driver for low-orbit space-based systems is the weight in orbit. Across this wide range of systems, weights and mission, space systems cost about $30,000 per kilogram.[31]

I can now apply the $30,000 per kilogram figure to my SBI system. Each interceptor might weigh 100 kilograms, with an additional 100 kilograms added to each to cover the cost of the satellite carrier and its sensors and support systems—a total weight in orbit of 200 kilograms per SBI. Each 10-interceptor satellite would weigh 2,000 kilograms and cost about $60 million. My whole system of 600 satellites would thus cost $36 billion. This estimate, as I have said, is consistent with other published values.

My bottom line for System A is $66 billion. This is comparable to the cost of redressing the Soviet COF advantage with wholly offensive responses. The defensive approach, of course, has the added advantage that it provides a meaningful level of damage limitation—i.e., it protects the people—should deterrence fail.

Possible Soviet Response to System A

Faced with losing their hard-won COF advantage in the mid-1990s, the Soviets would surely consider ways they could get it back in the late 1990s. Their two basic options are an upgraded offense and defense suppression. They might also consider expanding their own defenses. But as I stated earlier this would represent a de facto acceptance of the US-favored defensive deterrent relationship. The end result of a defensive arms race is the same deterrent relationship we hope to get.out of formal agreements. I will consider the defense suppression (survivability) issues separately. In this section I review possible Soviet offensive responses.

I see two forms of Soviet mid-term offensive response. The Soviets might simply build more of what they have today in order to overwhelm US defensive System A. Although hotly contested by SDI critics, I believe it unlikely that the Soviets could develop and deploy significant numbers of a totally new type of offense "responsive" to the initial defense before the year 2000.[32] They could, however, implement one form of responsive offense in the late 1990s—offensive system decoys. Decoy boosters, while feasible, do not seem to be a very promising response for cost reasons.[33] The GBI is designed to intercept the small warhead in space and it requires a sophisticated infrared sensor. It's relatively easy and cheap to imitate the warhead. However, it is costly and difficult to imitate the hot booster plume the SBI is designed to home in on.

To be effective, warhead decoys must be lightweight. As with satellites, the cost of any object launched into space is in direct relation to its weight.

Whether the Soviets simply add warheads to recover those the defense destroys or try a combination of added warheads and decoys, the cost to them is about the same. System A is designed to destroy 9,600 warheads—so that is the number the Soviets would have to add. Conversely, they could add only the warheads destroyed by the global defense and deploy decoys to negate the sovereign area defense. But the weight penalty imposed by the decoys is about the same as the weight of the 3,600 added warheads needed to overwhelm the GBI in System A. Either way, the Soviets would have to add about 10,000 warheads to recover their COF advantage.

How many rubles the 10,000 new Soviet warheads might cost is unknown. But it is reasonable to assume that the Soviet Union isn't any more efficient at building ICBMs and warheads than the United States. We need only ask what it would cost the United States to add 10,000 warheads to our arsenal. As I observed at the beginning of this chapter, the cheapest US missile warheads are the heavily MIRVed MX systems—at $20 million apiece. It's reasonable to assume, therefore, that the Soviet offensive response to System A might cost them the equivalent of 9600 × $20 million = $192 billion.

Defense System B

We must now ask two questions. First, what must the defense do to redress to Soviet offensive response? Second, and more significantly, what US defensive move would best continue the trend toward elimination of ballistic missiles as instruments of national policy?

US System B could be deployed in the latter half of the 1990s to negate the Soviet responses to System A. To the global defense layer we might make two improvements. An additional 6,000 SBI interceptors, for a total of 12,000, would negate 6,000 of the new offensive warheads proliferated by the Soviets. Second, a series of low-earth-orbit sensor satellites—a Space Surveillance and Tracking System, or SSTS—would extend SBI capability so that they could intercept the cold warheads even after separation from the booster and bus. Of course, Soviet decoys might also be able to confuse and complicate this ability.

System B would also include major additions to the sovereign area defenses designed to counter the Soviet warhead decoys. When a decoy or warhead reenters the earth's atmosphere, it slows down due to atmospheric drag—a lighter decoy slows down a lot more rapidly than a heavy decoy. If we can measure this difference, we can "filter" the warheads from the decoys. This atmospheric filtering was the main reason for developing the Sprint system in the 1960s—as a way to counter decoys. Thus, inside the atmosphere, or endo-atmospheric, defense defeats decoys. The 1960s Sprint had poor sensors and limited battle management capabilities, so it served only as a point defense. But the SDI program is developing a new technology that could make an endo-atmospheric area defense feasible.

By the late 1990s an endo-atmospheric GBI Defense Interceptor will be deployable. These "endo-GBIs" would rely not only on the airborne infrared sensors used by ERIS, but also on a small mobile ground-based radar. The combination of new sensors and improved endo-GBI interceptors could enable it to cover an area several hundred kilometers across—thus endo-GBI would be an area defense system, not a point defense. Like the exo-GBI, the endo-GBI would not destroy its warhead target with a nuclear explosion but would use kinetic energy to do the job. In the case of endo-GBI, it might not actually hit the warhead target, but might scatter a small cloud of shrapnel in its path.

To preserve the COF reduction won by System A, System B must destroy the additional 6,000 warheads added by the Soviets and undo the effects of the Soviet decoys. As I stated above, an additional 6,000 SBIs would take care of the additional Soviet warheads. But what about the decoys?

Remembering that we are trying to set the stage against further Soviet countermoves, it makes sense to handle the decoys in two ways. By enabling the SBI to hit warheads in space we might bring up to 40 percent of the absentee SBI units into play in the 30 minutes of midcourse flight. Although most of these would be confused by the Soviet decoys, they might be able to stop 500 more of the Soviet warheads, and 5,000 of the Soviet decoys. Like the SBI, exo-ground-based intercepters would only kill one warhead for every ten objects hit. Nonetheless, it makes sense to add exo-GBI interceptors—6,000 of which would bring the total exo-GBI arsenal to 10,000 interceptors. Between exo-GBI and SBI they would kill only 1,500 or so warheads—and at an unfavorable cost exchange with the offense. The reason for this short-term unfavorable deployment will become clear when I talk about the final defensive deployment—System C. In System C we will include systems to discriminate between warheads and decoys in space.

In order to bring us back to the point System A got us to, endo-GBI must stop 2,000 warheads which the other systems missed. Unfortunately, endo-GBI are more expensive than exo-GBI and less efficient, because each site covers a smaller area. Each endo-GBI would cost about $4.5 million to deploy and maintain for ten years, 50 percent more than the exo-GBI unit cost. Moreover, the Soviets might target in such a way as to exhaust some endo-GBI sites and leave others untouched. For this reason, I believe that only 70 percent of the endo-GBI in the system would hit their targets, as opposed to 90 percent for exo-GBI.[34] Thus, 3000 endo-GBI and their associated radars would complete our counter to the Soviet decoys.

Table 4 (page 184) also shows my cost estimates for System B. The defensive response to a Soviet offensive deployment costing the equivalent of $192 billion is $82 billion. Of course, these estimates are uncertain, but they suggest that System B meets the cost-effectiveness at the margin requirement quite handily.

Possible Soviet Response to System B

As I consider actions and counteractions in the first decade of the next century, my crystal ball becomes quite murky. Unfortunately, much of the public debate over strategic defenses has focused on this "science fiction" era.[35] I have no intention of repeating here the esoteric arguments which run a wide range of possible countermeasures and counter-countermeasures. But I do think the reader would benefit from a single example of far-term Soviet countermeasures to defenses and one possible US response. I've chosen examples which pop up frequently in public arguments so that this discussion might continue to have value in the future.

New Soviet offensive systems in the 2000s must get through the three defensive layers I described previously—two sovereign area defense layers and one global. There are, of course, suggestions on how to do this. Among the most discussed countermeasures to a global defense is the so-called "fast-burn booster" or FBB.[36] A FBB would finish thrusting its warhead payload while still within the upper reaches of the atmosphere—out of harm's way from space-based defenses which generally cannot operate in the atmosphere. By way of a working assumption, I'll assume that the Soviets would add 10,000 FBB warheads to recover the advantages that US defensive Systems A and B denied them.

How much would 10,000 FBB warheads cost the Soviets, and when could they get them? In 1983 the US Government Fletcher Study suggested that the Soviets could not get substantial numbers of FBBs until after the year 2000.[37] FBBs would be small ICBMs—probably single-warhead systems.[38] Thus, the Soviets would need 10,000 new boosters along with associated basing. To ensure survivability and maximize the ability to penetrate global defenses, these new systems should also be mobile.[39] The United States has no experience with small mobile ICBMs, but has designed such a system in the form of the proposed Midgetman. These missiles have been estimated to be very expensive—each Midgetman warhead would cost close to $100 million to deploy.[40] The FBB is at least as sophisticated as the Midgetman, so there is no reason to believe it would be any less expensive. The Soviet response to System B could well cost the equivalent of $900 billion—a cost comparable to the entire Soviet strategic offensive arsenal to date!

Concepts for US System C

Much of the SDI program addresses systems like the fast-burn booster (FBB). Possible FBB responses take two forms: defensive systems which can reach into the upper atmosphere to stop the FBB before it burns out; or systems for discriminating warheads from decoys in space.

Laser defensive weapons—either based in space or on the ground—are one way to stop the FBB while they are still in the atmosphere. Ground-based lasers would use relay mirrors in space to direct the killing laser energy to the FBB. Properly selected lasers can penetrate into the upper atmosphere to burn holes in the FBB or crack the rocket casing. Kilotons of paper have been wasted in arguments between SDI critics and proponents over the feasibility and cost of this response to the FBB. Particularly stressing to the laser approach would be a mass launch of FBB from a small region on the surface.[41]

Another solution to the FBB problem would be to deploy systems which can "interactively" discriminate warheads from decoys in space. If we could reliably discriminate the warheads, the SBI and GBI systems deployed in System B would be adequate to stop the entire 10,000 new FBB warheads after the booster has burned out and fallen away.

Interactive discrimination involves actively probing each potential threat object. Based on the response of the probed object, we can determine whether it's a real warhead. Directed energy, of which the laser is one form, is a good way to probe objects. We could also use a different form of directed energy than a laser—the neutral particle beam—for interactive discrimination. Lasers focus light—much as a magnifying glass can focus sunlight to burn holes in objects. A particle beam fires atoms or pieces of atoms at an object. Particle beams are known popularly as "atom smashers." Electric power accelerates individual atoms to nearly the speed of light. At these high energies the particles can penetrate deep inside an object. With enough particles, this could melt the target's internal mechanism. A smaller number of particles can disrupt sensitive electronics. But even a few particles can cause the target to emit radiation. The heavier the target, the more radiation gets released. If we measure the amount of radiation, we can translate that into how much the object weighs. Heavy objects can be assumed to be real warheads; light objects would be decoys which the defense could ignore.

How many neutral particle beam discriminators and associated sensors would be needed and how complicated are they? The SDI program plans a neutral particle beam and sensor experiment in the early 1990s to verify that the interactive discrimination scheme is feasible. This experiment will weigh about 20,000 kilograms and cost $700 million, but it is far from a deployable system. Nonetheless, very rough estimates of the number and features of a neutral particle beam discrimination system exist.[42] Approximately 50 space-based beam systems—including several hundred radiation sensors and associated survivability features—could be deployed between 2005 and 2010. An upper limit to the weight of each beam device is 100,000 kilograms. The sensor weights are negligible—a few hundred kilograms each. Using my rule of thumb for space system costs, this constellation would cost $50 \times 100,000$ kg $\times$ $30,000/kg = $150 billion.

As I discussed earlier, MaRV warheads might be able to defeat the endo-GBI systems. At this early time in endo-GBI system development we cannot know whether a non-nuclear kinetic energy interceptor will be capable enough to strike a maneuvering warhead inside the atmosphere. However, if the endo-GBI interceptor were equipped with a small nuclear warhead, its lethal radius would be large enough so that even a MaRV warhead would be out of luck.[43] The primary cost to retrofit non-nuclear endo-GBI with nuclear warheads would be the cost of those warheads—which I set at an upper limit of $5 million per warhead. I thus estimate that the United States could retrofit the entire endo-GBI force of 3,000 warheads to counter MaRVs for $15 billion.

I conclude that the $900 billion Soviet FBB force might be countered with about $165 billion of US defensive upgrades—a cost-exchange ratio favoring the defense by more than 5:1. Of course, this is only one scenario. SDI critics have proposed many other countermeasures. But the FBB is always at the top of the list. My "back of the envelope" calculation—the best anyone can do 20 years before the fact—certainly suggests that the defense could enjoy a very large cost-exchange advantage over offensive countermeasures well into the 21st century.

Can the United States afford these three generations of strategic defense? If so, would this require that we severely cut back our conventional expenditures? If the Soviets try to engage us in this offense-defense arms race, it certainly seems that the $1 trillion-plus price tag for their offensive moves is prohibitive. What about the approximately $300 billion cost to the United States for my Systems A, B and C? The United States currently spends about 15 percent of its defense budget on strategic forces—or about $45 billion per year. Between the years 1990 and 2010—during which my three defensive systems would be deployed—we might expect $900 billion to be spent by the United States on strategic forces if current trends continue.[44] In this context, my proposed defensive deployment is certainly affordable, and indeed a bargain!

Table 4 lists costs and numbers for each element in US Systems A, B, and C, as well as information on Soviet counters. Figure 13 shows how each system might operate.

Table 4. System Descriptions and Soviet Responses

US System A (1993-1997)

Components	*Costs*
Global Defense (SBI)	
6,000 Interceptors/600 Satellite Carriers	
($6 Million per Interceptor)	$36 Billion
4 Boost Surveillance and Track Satellites	
($2 Billion per Satellite)	$8 Billion
Sovereign Area Defense (GBI)	
4,000 Exo-atmospheric Interceptors	$12 Billion
($3 Million per Interceptor)	

20 Airborne Optical Sensor Planes ($500 Million per Airplane)	$10 Billion
Total Cost for System A	$66 Billion

Soviet Response to US System A (1995-2000)

Components	*Costs*
ICBM Proliferation (SS-18 Equivalents) 9,600 New ICBM Warheads ($20 Million per Warhead)	$192 Billion
Total Cost: Soviet Response to System A	$192 Billion

US System B (1997-2000)

Components	*Costs*
Global Defense (SBI) 6,000 Interceptors/600 Satellite Carriers ($6 Million per Interceptor)	$36 Billion
10 Space Surveillance Satellites ($1 Billion per Satellite)	$10 Billion
Sovereign Area Defense (GBI) 6,000 Exo-atmospheric Interceptors ($3 Million per Interceptor)	$18 Billion
3,000 Endo-atmospheric Interceptors ($4.5 Million per Interceptor)	$13.5 Billion
30 Radars/30 Mobile Radar Sites ($150 Million per Radar Site)	$4.5 Billion
Total Cost for US System B	$82 Billion

Soviet Response to US System B (2000-2005)

Components	*Cost*
10,000 Fast Burn Booster ICBMs—Single Warhead ($90 Million per Mobile Booster)	$900 Billion
Total Cost: Soviet Response to System B	$900 Billion

US System C (2005-2010)

Components	*Cost*
Global Defense (Interactive Discrimination) 50 Neutral Particle Beam Satellites ($3 Billion per Satellite/Sensor)	$150 Billion

Sovereign Area Defense (Nuclear-Armed Endo-atmospheric)
   3,000 Retrofit Interceptors $15 Billion
      ($5 Million per Retrofit)

Total Cost for US System C $165 Billion

Who Will Guard the Guards?

What if the Soviets reject direct offensive responses, concentrating instead on suppressing the defenses? In this way they might preserve their current offensive forces' ability to penetrate. They could build their defense suppression systems under the guise of building "defensive" systems. For example, if both superpowers chose to deploy large global defenses, space would be "co-occupied." If our defensive system were to be vulnerable, the situation might be unstable. As a prelude to a first strike, one could use its "defensive" system to knock out the other's system. This instability might actually encourage a preemptive move during a crisis for fear the other would get in the first blow. This possible defensive instability is a new element in the 1990s SDI debate—possibly the only new strategic factor. It is a central feature in both US and Soviet SDI critics' arguments.[45] It is, nevertheless, specious.

Military co-occupancy of an international medium is not new—even with strategic nuclear systems. Military forces have co-occupied the seas for millennia. Both Allied and Soviet nuclear submarines—the mainstay of Western deterrent forces—occupy the same oceans. Now, both sides' submarines are in principle vulnerable to the other's naval forces. However, we consider the situation stable because it is sufficiently difficult to locate and destroy each others' submarines.

Space operations would have many similarities to submarine warfare—despite SDI critics' attempts to deny this analogy.[46] Rather than discussing highly sensitive submarine and anti-submarine warfare, I believe another analogy—World War I air operations—will illustrate the principles.

At the start of World War I both sides used aircraft for only two purposes. They spied on each other, and carried messages.

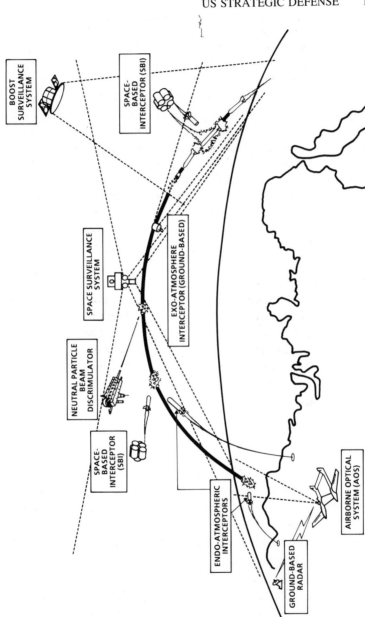

Figure 13. Proposed US Missile Defense Systems A, B, and C

Basically, that's all military spacecraft do in the 1990s. The situation quickly changed in World War I. Airplanes soon became useful for strafing the enemy—stopping supplies and killing front-line troops. Not surprisingly, each side came to object to the strafing, the spying and the message carrying—so they shot at opposing airplanes from the ground and from their own aircraft. Air warfare had begun. If I apply the logic advanced by SDI critics to this situation, World War I experience should have ended for all time the role of airplanes in war. If combatants were going to shoot at airplanes, these would clearly be useless—and should be banned. After all, the air is transparent so that the enemy could see the airplanes at great distances, and they travel in straight lines—turning only slowly, by comparison with a horse, for example. Finally, planes were delicate instruments, made of sealing wax and wire and carrying gallons of explosive fuel. A single bullet could easily destroy a plane.

Airpower advocates in World War I must certainly have heard these arguments—and quickly proved them wrong. Airplanes were made more maneuverable and camouflaged, becoming far more difficult to see and to track. Armor plate was added to vulnerable points—not the least of which was the battle management system, or pilot. Industry learned to mass produce the planes cheaply, so that even if many were shot down, more could easily be bought. Finally, the pilots recognized that they could arm their aircraft and shoot back. These technologies and tactics have made aircraft sufficiently survivable to become a mainstay of many nations' military capabilities.[47] During the 1950s—and beyond—they have been the predominant basis of nuclear deterrence despite their vulnerability. The same technologies and tactics which made aircraft militarily survivable can and are being applied to military space systems.

I will consider three types of defense-suppression attack. In order to decide whether the offense or defense wins, I will use a cost-exchange criteria. If it costs less to preserve the strategic change in COF produced by the defense than to restore it with defense suppression—I consider the situation stable. The three forms of defense supression are:

1. Attempts to deny deployment—that is, by shooting down each defensive element as it's put into space.

2. Attrition attacks over long periods—slowly knocking down the system after it's been put into place.

3. Sudden attacks as a prelude to an offensive nuclear strike. In that instance, the offense need only blow a hole in the defense through which to fire offensive forces.

There are numerous discussions of space system survivability against determined suppression attacks given elsewhere, so I will only illustrate the general features of such an engagement here.[48] I consider an attack against System A from the most potent defense suppression means likely to be available in the 1990s. The Soviets and Western SDI critics cite ground-based nuclear-armed ABMs as the most likely and potent defense suppression means.[49] The Soviet Union already has these systems in place around Moscow and could easily mass produce them in the 1990s.[50]

In order for Soviet defense supression to be effective it must, at a minimum, restore the COF advantage enjoyed prior to initial defense deployment. In order for them to choose defense suppression, its advantages must be weighed against the cost of alternatives. For example, if the Soviets could buy back their COF advantage with offensive means more cheaply than with defense suppression that would be their favored approach. Against System A, as I have shown, it would cost the Soviets about $190 billion to defeat it with offensive proliferation. Of course, suppressing the space-based portion doesn't do the whole job—the ground-based defenses would still be in place. I thus prorate the space-based portion of the Soviet offensive counter as costing $120 billion.

As I discussed earlier in this chapter, space-based, kinetic-kill, vehicle-carrier satellite might cost about $60 million. It is reasonable to assume that a Soviet nuclear-armed ABM costs slightly more than my baseline non-nuclear endo-GBI, or $6 million each. It would appear to be a bargain for the Soviets to take out a defensive satellite, but this assumes that the satellite does nothing to ensure its survivability. As designed, these $60 million satellites would include many survivability features.

First, the defensive satellites could include hardening to make sure that nothing but a near hit with a nuclear weapon might knock it out. Today, our satellites are "soft." A one-megaton blast might kill satellites within thousands of kilometers. But there is no reason why future satellites could not be at least as hard as their warhead targets—in which case a nuclear warhead would have to detonate within a few kilometers to kill the satellite.[51]

How many nuclear-armed ABMs are needed to kill a hardened satellite? If the Soviet ABMs are ''dumb,'' in that they cannot track an object after they are fired but must hope that it hasn't moved, all the prospective target needs to do to survive is to move out of the way. It is easy to move a few kilometers—out of lethal range—between the time the ABM is fired and when it gets to its preset position. To move a few kilometers in 60 seconds or so would take fuel equal to only about two percent of the satellite's weight. Each $60 million satellite would be designed to carry enough fuel for ten maneuvers. With this capability, the cost exchange between satellite and ABM is evened up to 1:1.

If Soviet ABMs can home in on a maneuvering target—an expensive proposition for a heavy nuclear interceptor which could well double its cost—the satellite target must try something else. If it releases a cheap lightweight decoy, it could confuse the attacker. The satellite can wait until the last second to throw out the decoy and thus the attacker is unlikely to be able to discriminate between it and a decoy. A credible decoy could weigh 1 percent or less than the satellite. Each could carry 30 or more decoys. If the Soviets choose non-nuclear systems like the exo-GBI—at $3 million a copy—instead of expensive nuclear-armed ABMs, that would gain them little. Since the real target doesn't have to move very far to get out of range after it releases a decoy, it would have fuel for dozens of maneuvers. In either case, the combination of survivability and maneuvering would buy the defense a cost exchange advantage over the offense of about 2:1 for a one-on-one engagement.

But the defense hasn't exhausted its means of survivability. If the Soviets fired enough ABMs to get through all of the decoys and follow the maneuvering satellite, the satellite itself is still armed with its kinetic-kill vehicles, and it could expend some of these to defend itself. Since each satellite has ten interceptors, the Soviets would have to fire at least ten of those at each target—after they got through the decoys. To handle a satellite and its decoys might well take hundreds of ABMs and the cost exchange could favor the defense by factors of ten to twenty. There are other means the satellite could use, such as jamming and deception, which could add even more to its survivability. History has already shown us that it is not easy to kill a moving object which is defended by decoys, the ability to maneuver, and the means to shoot back. It took the North Vietnamese many hundreds of SAMs to shoot down B-52s defended like that in the Vietnam war.

I can now figure how expensive it would be for the Soviets to winnow out our defense, either during or after deployment, since attrition attacks are one-on-one engagements. For the Soviets to knock down 600 satellites might cost them $400-800 billion. Defense suppression appears much less appealing than offensive proliferation in this case.

A much different case would be Soviet interest in blowing a hole in the system rather than knocking it down. Because they wouldn't worry about the absentee satellites, they only need to destroy the 90 satellites over the Soviet Union when they decide to strike. Of course, the remaining satellites would still be in place to stop SLBMs. Moreover, the Soviets must be able to coordinate an essentially instantaneous defense suppression and offensive strike. If stretched out more than 5 minutes, new defensive satellites would orbit into place and the defense suppression would be for nothing. To knock down the 90 satellites would require 20,000 or more ABMs at a cost of $60-180 billion. Moreover, since boost phase lasts more than five minutes for some Soviet systems, they would have to shoot down some of the SBI outside the territorial areas of the Soviet Union. This defense suppression approach is comparable in cost to doing the job with offensive proliferation alone. But it also has the added complexity of a battle management problem at least as stressing as that the defense would face, with even more uncertainty for the offense.

For the Soviets, the defense suppression route could itself have a negative impact on their COF calculation. To refer once again to their COF equation, I feel they must multiply the probability of penetrating the defense by the probability that the defense suppression will work. For example, if the Soviets judged that their defense suppression had a 30 percent chance of succeeding, that would remove their COF advantage just as surely as a 65 percent effective defense. The necessity of negating a defense as a prelude before an attack further strengthens deterrence and weakens Soviet advantages.

Although the "what if?" game becomes much harder the farther I peer into the future, two longer term defense suppression programs warrant discussion. "Space mines" are another favorite of SDI critics.[52] A space mine is a small device which sidles up to a space-based defensive satellite, stays with it and homes in for the kill upon command when the aggressor wishes to strike. Space mines don't exist today, but they could well be developed as a defense suppression means against defensive System B.

What would a space mine cost, and how well would it work? Basically, a space mine is a sophisticated version of the defensive SBI. It is sophisticated because it must stay with the small SBI carrier satellites. Space mine enthusiasts—invariably critics of SDI—believe that space mines are cheap, at about $3 million each. Ironically, the same folks who cite this cost insist that a strategic defense, which they acknowledge could have as few as 10,000 SBI, would cost "trillions." Including guidance and control functions, as well as ground support, I can't imagine a space mine weighing less than 500 kilograms and thus costing less than $15 million. The space mine must maneuver to follow the SBI satellite, if for no other reason than to adjust its orbit to make up for drag caused by the residual atmosphere and solar wind. *All* satellites maneuver for this reason. The space mine's small rocket firings will give it away—thus it is not like the invisible sea mines it is named for. Once the SBKKV sees that it is being followed, it could simply launch a decoy and slip away. It would be impossible for the Soviets to build enough space mines to follow all of the SBKKVs and decoys. Space mines are not, therefore, a serious defense suppression threat.

In the long term, the Soviets might try to use directed-energy weapons to suppress the defense—by that time defensive System C. For example, they might use ground-based lasers to knock down weapons and sensors in space.[53] These lasers require some time to knock down each satellite and much more time to degrade a system. This approach is useful, therefore, purely as an attrition attack. It is unclear whether it will be cheaper to launch laser shielding into space than it would be to use the ground-based laser to burn this shielding away. But it would be silly for the United States to tolerate such attacks. By any reading of international law, destruction of sovereign military assets in international areas is an act of war.[54] The United States would be fully justified in taking whatever actions are necessary to stop the laser attacks. Considering that the ground-based laser would be a mile-long fixed facility, it would surely be much easier to put it out of commission than any asset in space.

*   *   *

This brief technical analysis shows that strategic defenses could well meet the necessary requirements. Unfortunately, the decision on whether to move to a defense-reliant deterrent will not be made on whether they meet these requirements—although that will certainly be a necessary condition. Emotional and political arguments will be far more important. The proponents of MAD are united and dedicated, while Western advocates of warfighting strategies are less emotional—but they are also firmly entrenched in the defense intellectual and bureaucratic community. The Soviet Union is adept at using politics to achieve arms control agreements which could foreclose any moves toward defense-reliant deterrence. The new Soviet leadership has learned the value of good public relations and pleasantries when they desire a one-sided arms control deal. As my analysis has shown, space is a key to a successful strategic defense. If the Soviets and the "useful idiots" in the West, as Lenin once called them, succeed in forging an arms control deal to keep defensive weapons from space, all will be lost. The Soviet Union has already benefited greatly from those in Congress and in the public who have succeeded in slowing progress on the SDI and blocking some vital capabilities, such as new heavy-lift launch capabilities.

But the final decision is up to the American people. They must consider the alternatives and choose whether they want their security based on trust of the Soviet Union and weapons of mass destruction, or on a new way which relies on neither.

EPILOGUE

In the past three years, the world has certainly turned "upside down." The Cold War is generally regarded to be over, with monolithic communism assigned to the dust bin of history. In the years ahead numerous scholars undoubtedly will address the cause of its collapse and try to explain the suddenness of that collapse.

Needless to say, this author would attribute much of the pressure behind these changes to the Strategic Defense Initiative. The basic thesis of this book is that SDI intended to drive the Soviets away from strategic offensive strategies in particular and away from quantitative strategic paradigms in general. It appears that SDI did just this. By demonstrating that the Soviets' hard won correlation-of-forces advantages could be cheaply wiped out, SDI started the ball rolling. But, by further raising the specter of new, unpredictable space-based offensive capabilities in the hands of their adversaries, SDI convinced the Soviets that the chances of success in a future arms competition would be extremely low. Once the Soviets understood these realities, their military or quantitative basis for grand strategy vaporized. With that basic assumption of Soviet power gone, many other Soviet assumptions evaporated as well.

The technical breakthrough which made SDI manifestly cost effective at the margin is the so-called "brilliant pebble" developed by the Lawrence Livermore National Laboratory. This kinetic energy interceptor—consisting of a small (50-kilogram) self-contained satellite with a very large, on-board computing capability and wide field-of-view sensor—is estimated to cost at most a few million dollars per copy. Thus each interceptor is considerably cheaper than the warhead or missile it would go after, and much cheaper than the anti-satellite weapon designed to destroy it.

With SDI having succeeded "brilliantly" in dispelling the Soviet military calculations supporting the Cold War, the obvious issue now is the future of the program. I see three possible directions:

First, although the Soviet Union has agreed to move away from nuclear offensive-based strategies, over 10,000 modern warheads remain in its arsenals. Furthermore, those numbers are *not* being significantly reduced.[1] Until these weapons are removed, the real danger remains of a resurgent and virulent Soviet (or nationalist) government in the USSR that might use them to threaten others. In this eventuality, SDI could serve as a lever to force continued reductions in these arms, regardless of future Soviet Government intentions.

The United States and its allies won the war with Iraq, a nation which used medium-range SCUD missiles against the allies and Israel and earlier had used chemical weapons against Iran and Kurdish rebels. The allies were able to destroy much of Iraq's nuclear, chemical, biological, and missile capabilities. Despite these allied successes, Iraq is a case-in-point of the threat represented by a small or middle-size power which possesses the means and will to develop and use weapons of mass destruction. A second approach for the SDI program would be to reorient toward countering these potential threats— either as an inducement for nations such as Iraq to not develop such capabilities, or a means to counter their use.[2]

Finally, SDI has already proven to be a fertile ground for developing technologies with wide-ranging economic and military implications. So a third potential future focus for SDI might be as a means to develop new technologies with broad military application.

While the first two rationales are compelling enough, the third holds a different, long-range potential. On 20 July 1989, President Bush set the United States on a renewed course to explore and ultimately inhabit the Solar System. He later directed that the Departments of Defense and Energy play major roles in this Space Exploration Initiative (SEI).[3] Space exploration could be the wellspring of economic prosperity for the 21st century, providing unlimited access to resources and non-polluting sources of energy.[4] Other industrialized nations, such as Japan, have targeted these benefits and show every sign of giving the United States a run for its money.[5]

SDI is relevant to SEI for two reasons. First, many of the technologies which could make US space exploration both affordable and fast-paced enough to stay ahead of its economic competitors have come from SDI programs.[6] Second, SDI seems to provide a successful model for how to approach new, technologically challenging programs. By providing large amounts of money for technology development, and forcing alternative system architectures to compete, as in SDI directed-energy versus kinetic-energy architectures, an affordable program emerges. Whereas initial cost estimates for deploying an SDI system were as high as $500 billion, estimates in 1990 were about an order of magnitude lower.[7] The enforced period of intense technology development and architectural competition provides an outstanding opportunity for faster, cheaper, and better ideas to emerge. It is no accident that SEI resembles SDI in approach.[8]

A second potential long-range product of SDI was alluded to earlier in this book. In the likely military scenarios of the next decade and beyond, such as the 1990–91 Middle Eastern crisis, there might be a role for space-based force application capabilities. By applying precise offensive capabilities, perhaps through a variant of the brilliant pebbles kinetic energy device or space-based directed energy systems capable of penetrating the atmosphere, aggressive actions by nations such as Iraq against Kuwait could be countered within minutes, instead of the months needed to position ground and air forces. Furthermore, the direct risk to US lives would be considerably lower. While such systems are not currently under development, National Space Policy states that they could be developed should the need arise.[9]

So perhaps the most promising new role for SDI—not envisioned at its birth in 1983—would be as incubator or catalyst for space technologies essential to economic competitiveness, and for national security force projection. As the decade of the 1990s unfolds, this prospect offers hope for future security, stability, and peace even as the nations of the world bend to the sober and dangerous task of bringing justice and order to a turbulent world.

NOTES

Introduction: The Elements in the Strategic Debate

1. Robert S. McNamara, *Blundering into Disaster* (New York: Pantheon, 1986), p. 96. McNamara says, "Mutual assured destruction—the vulnerability of each superpower to the awesome destructive power of nuclear weapons—is not a policy at all. It is a fact of life."

2. Bernard Brodie, editor, *The Absolute Weapon* (New York: Harcourt Brace and Co., 1946).

3. The Chinese General Sun Tzu, outlined circa 400 B.C. a strategy predicated on avoiding battle by confounding the enemy's plans. See chapter 3.

4. Major General I. Anureyev, "Determining the Correlation of Forces in Terms of Nuclear Weapons," *Voyennaya Mysl* (*Military Thought*), No. 6, 1967.

5. Stephen M. Meyer, "Soviet Strategic Programs and the U.S. SDI," *Survival*, November-December 1985, pp. 274-292.

6. Zbigniew Brzezinski, *Game Plan* (Boston: The Atlantic Monthly Press, 1986) pp. 147-148. There is also growing recognition on the part of the US military of the conventional importance of space. See, for example, Major Arthur L. Bennett, Jr., *Command of the Aerospace: Convergence of Theory and Technology in Shaping an Aerospace Force for 2025* (Maxwell AFB, AL: Air University Press, AU-ARI-86-8, August 1986).

7. J.F.C. Fuller, *Armament and History* (New York: Scribners, 1945), p. 7.

8. Albert Wohlstetter, *Commentary*, 1983.

9. Kinetic energy weapons kill a target by striking it. At the relative velocities involved in space operations, kinetic energy of motion is much larger than any conventional explosive—and even approaches nuclear energy levels. A ten-ton rock dropped from lunar orbit would strike the earth with almost a kiloton of kinetic energy. Kinetic energy

space weapons can be no more complex than an air-to-air type missile mounted on a satellite. Directed energy weapons, in comparison, fire energy in the form of light (lasers) or atomic particles (particle beam). The beams travel at or near the speed of light.

10. For example, the X-ray laser. The nuclear explosion powers the laser. This weapon has the advantage that it takes the immense power of a nuclear weapon and directs a portion of it in a particular direction. The "brightness" of an X-ray laser can be very high. However, nuclear directed-energy weapons are destroyed in firing and are inherently single-shot devices. See US Congress, Office of Technology Assessment, *Ballistic Missile Defense Technologies* (Washington, DC: US Government Printing Office, OTA-ISC-254, September 1985), pp. 152-153.

1. Vulnerability-Based Nuclear Deterrence

1. Carl Sagan, "The Case Against SDI," *Discover*, September, 1985, pp. 67-75.

1. Leo Szilard wrote a memorandum to President Roosevelt in March 1945. The letter never reached the President owing to Roosevelt's sudden death. The full text of Szilard's letter is in the *Bulletin of the Atomic Scientists*, Volume 3, 1947, pp. 351-353.

3. Whether Robert Oppenheimer actually quoted the Shiva statement is unclear. A discussion of the physicist's emotional reaction to the Trinity test is given in Peter Goodchild, *J. Robert Oppenheimer: Shatterer of Worlds* (Boston: Houghton Mifflin, 1981), pp. 148-164.

4. *Bulletin of the Atomic Scientists*, 10 December 1945, p. 1.

5. *New York Times*, "Atom Bomb Defense Indicated by Navy," 12 October 1945, pp. 1, 5.

6. *New York Times*, "Scientist Group Hits Atomic Bill," 19 October 1945, p. 2.

7. Although statements cleared ahead of time do not call current US strategy MAD, which it is in fact not, President Reagan and other

officials' off-the-cuff remarks frequently slip. For example, in his interview with *New York Times* correspondents on 11 February 1985 he said, "The only program we have is MAD—Mutual Assured Destruction. And why don't we have MAS—Mutual Assured Security instead?" For this and similar quotes see *Star Wars Quotes* compiled by the Arms Control Association (Washington, DC: The Arms Control Association, 1986).

8. Thucydides, *The Peloponnesian War*, translated by Rex Warner (New York: Penguin Books, 1972), pp. 400-408.

9. Giulio Douhet, *Command of the Air*, translated by Dino Ferrari (New York: Coward-McCann Inc., 1942).

10. Ibid., p. 196.

11. The debate prior to World War II on whether Britain would rely on an offensive bomber deterrent or on air defenses is similar in many ways to the 1980s debate on ballistic missile defense. The principal protagonists in Britain were Prime Minister Stanley Baldwin, who was concerned with cost and pacifist sentiment, and Winston Churchill, an obscure member of parliament at the time who was concerned with Germany's offensive buildup. Churchill's victory in the debate was crucial to Britain in the war. An excellent review of the controversy is given by Benson D. Adams, "Strategy and the First Strategic Defense Initiative," *Naval War College Review*, November-December 1985, pp. 50-58.

12. John Foster Dulles, Secretary of State, speech made before the Council on Foreign Relations, New York, on 12 January 1954, *Department of State Bulletin*, 25 January 1954.

13. The fact that Dulles's "New Look" was a continuation of US strategic policy and the motivations for the initiative in 1954 are reviewed by Samuel F. Wells, Jr., "The Origins of Massive Retaliation," *Political Science Quarterly*, Spring 1981, pp. 21-52.

14. Bernard Brodie, "Part I: The Weapon," in *The Absolute Weapon*, edited by Bernard Brodie (New York: Harcourt, Brace and Co., 1946), pp. 21-107.

15. Bernard Brodie wrote an introduction to a current edition of Karl von Clausewitz, *On War*, edited and translated by Michael Howard and Peter Paret (Princeton: Princeton University Press, 1976), pp. 45-58. In this introduction, he touted this classic work's value, but also suggested that its warfighting precepts were not relevant to nuclear issues.

16. B.H. Liddell Hart, *The Revolution in Warfare* (New Haven: Yale University Press, 1947).

17. Sir John Slessor, *Strategy for the West* (New York: William Morrow and Company, 1954).

18. Winston Churchill's "Balance of Terror" speech was his last to the British House of Commons. It is particularly significant in that it marked the first official adoption of MAD by a major power. The speech itself covered a policy expounded in a British Defence Ministry White Paper prepared in 1954. The Churchill speech was a fitting legacy for him and can be found in *Churchill Speaks* (New York: Chelsea House, 1980), pp. 966-971, Robert Rhodes James, editor.

19. Pierre Gallois, *The Balance of Terror: Strategy for the Nuclear Age* (Boston: Houghton-Mifflin, 1961).

20. The strategists of the late 1950s and early 1960s worked during the "Golden Age" of deterrence theory. Many of these theorists served as senior government officials in later administrations. A representative list and some key works are: Albert Wohlstetter, "The Delicate Balance of Terror," *Foreign Affairs,* January 1959, pp. 211-234; Henry Kissinger, "Force and Diplomacy in the Nuclear Age," *Foreign Affairs,* April 1956, pp. 349-366; Herman Kahn, *On Thermonuclear War* (Princeton: Princeton University Press, 1960); Paul H. Nitze, "Atoms, Strategy and Policy," *Foreign Affairs,* January 1956, pp. 187-198; and Thomas Schelling, *Arms and Influence* (New Haven: Yale University Press, 1966).

21. Bertrand Russell, *Common Sense and Nuclear Warfare* (New York: Simon and Schuster, 1959), p. 30.

22. Lawrence Freedman, *The Evolution of Nuclear Strategy* (New York: St. Martin's Press, 1981), pp. 185-189.

23. For more than anyone could ever want to know about models of bargaining and crisis management, see Glen H. Snyder and Paul Diesing, *Conflict Among Nations* (Princeton: Princeton University Press, 1977), Chapters II and III, pp. 33-281.

24. Thomas Schelling, *Arms and Influence* (New Haven: Yale University Press, 1966).

25. Schelling's ideas were criticized, along with those of other deterrent strategists beginning in the mid-1960s. The critics tended to take leftist views and used considerable sarcasm to press their points. For example, Schelling's 1966 *Arms and Influence* ideas were referred to as "The Rationality of the Irrational" by Stephen Maxwell, "Rationality in Deterrence," *Adelphi Papers,* No. 50 (London: Institute for Strategic Studies, August 1968).

26. Graham T. Allison and Morton H. Halperin, *Bureaucratic Politics: A Paradigm and Some Policy Implications* (Washington, DC: Brookings Institution, 1972).

27. Herman Kahn, *On Thermonuclear War* (Princeton: Princeton University Press, 1960).

28. James R. Newmann, "Review of *On Thermonuclear War,*" *Scientific American,* March 1961, pp. 197-200.

29. *Los Angeles Times* reporter Robert Scheer interviewed Mr. T.K. Jones, Deputy Under Secretary of Defense, in the fall of 1981. He published portions of this interview in "U.S. Could Survive in Administration's View," *Los Angeles Times,* 16 January 1982. The Jones quote became a rallying cry for critics of Reagan administration policy. The book by Robert Scheer, *With Enough Shovels* (New York: Random House, 1982), pp. 18-26, illustrates the critical and sarcastic view the liberal/academic press took toward Jones's ideas.

30. Stanley L. Thompson and Stephen H. Schneider, "Nuclear Winter Revisited," *Foreign Affairs,* Summer 1986, pp. 981-1005.

31. In November, 1983, a group of scientists, among whom Carl Sagan is best known, announced the discovery of nuclear winter. (See Carl Sagan, "Nuclear Winter and Climatic Catastrophe: Some Policy Implications," *Foreign Affairs,* Winter 1983/84, pp. 357-392.) Sagan was quick to identify nuclear winter as a realization of Herman Kahn's "doomsday" machine—concluding that nuclear war could result in mankind's extinction. In particular, nuclear winter theory predicted that the Northern Hemisphere would be plunged into several months of exceedingly cold nights. Smoke from burning cities would block so much sunlight that summer temperatures could fall to well below freezing. The effect was supposed to spread, in time, to both hemispheres, killing most plant life, resulting in devastation of the ecosphere and possible extinction of mankind. Sagan also identified a nuclear threshold below which nuclear winter would not occur. Not surprisingly, this threshold, about 1000 warheads, was precisely that recommended by MAD theory.

Sagan was quick to promote the MAD solution—a drastic reduction in offensive *arrangements* to the MAD level. Nuclear winter rapidly became a driving force for the nuclear freeze and disarmament movements. By 1986, it was clear that the nuclear winter calculations were wrong—see Thompson Schneider's paper cited above. He concluded, "The temperature changes more closely describe a nuclear *'fall'* than a nuclear winter with the effects now being in the range of a one-week temperature drop of 20° F—insufficient to produce any of the effects postulated." Some US experts think Sagan's calculations were deliberately faked, and point to an unholy alliance between elements of the press and certain scientists. For example, Russell Sitz, "In From the Cold: 'Nuclear Winter' Melts Down," *The National*

Interest, Fall 1986, pp. 3-17, shows that, while rigorous calculations eroded nuclear winter's basis, the press progressively increased scientific exaggeration of its effects.

32. Carl F. Miller, *Assessment of Nuclear Weapons Requirements for Assured Destruction* (URS Research Corporation, 757-6, February 1970).

33. Lt. General Glenn Kent, USAF (Ret) granted me an interview on 31 July 1986. During this interview he gave me a formerly classified study which he had prepared in 1964 and which, he said, Robert McNamara had used as the basis for his assured destruction and damage-limiting assessments. Much of the material in this 195-page study, "A Summary Study of Strategic Offensive and Defensive Forces of the U.S. and USSR," prepared for the Director of Defense Research and Engineering, 8 September 1964, appeared in the 1965 Defense Department statement to the House Armed Services Committee.

34. US Congress, Office of Technology Assessment, *Ballistic Missile Defense Technologies* (Washington, DC: U.S. Government Printing Office, 1985), pp. 385-389.

35. Robert S. McNamara's statements to Congress during his tenure as Secretary of Defense mark a change in declared US deterrent strategy in favor of MAD. These statements progressively lower the requirements for assured destruction. In his statement to the House Armed Services Committee on 27 January 1964 McNamara said 50 million dead would suffice for assured destruction, or by my calculation about 25-35 percent of the population. In his statement a year later (18 February 1965) he explicitly stated as assured destruction one-third to one-fourth of the population and two-thirds of industrial capacity (p. 39). On 23 January 1967, before the Senate Armed Services and Appropriations Committees, he cited one-fifth to one-fourth (20-25 percent) population loss and one-half to two-thirds industrial loss as assured destruction goals (p. 39). In McNamara's last statement in 1968 he maintained the same population loss numbers, but had lowered industrial loss to one-half (p. 50). In this document he explicitly said he was not sure whether 10 percent population loss was sufficient to deter the Soviet Union.

36. Robert S. McNamara and Hans A. Bethe, "Reducing the Risk of Nuclear War," *Atlantic Monthly,* July 1985, pp. 43-51.

37. Herman Kahn, *On Thermonuclear War,* p. 132.

38. Nevil Schute, *On the Beach* (New York: William Morrow, 1957).

39. In 1984 ABC Television prepared a made-for-TV movie, *The Day After*, depicting a nuclear attack on Kansas. Although there were intense Department of Defense public affairs preparations to counter the negative impacts of this movie, negative impacts did not materialize.

40. Pierre Gallois, *The Balance of Terror*, p. 19.

41. National Commission on Space, *Pioneering the Space Frontier* (New York: Bantam, 1986), p. 185.

42. Herman Kahn, *On Thermonuclear War*, p. 132.

43. Robert S. Gottfried, *The Black Death* (New York: The Free Press/ Macmillan, 1983), pp. 77, 102-103, 129-133.

44. Civil Defense Preparedness Agency, *Information Bulletin No 307* (Washington, DC: US Government Printing Office, 10 March 1979), p. 16.

45. Jennifer Leaning and Matthew Leighton, "The World According to FEMA," *Bulletin of the Atomic Scientists*, June-July 1983, pp. 38-39.

46. Testimony of General David Jones, in "Strategic Weapons Proposals," *Hearings Before the Committee on Foreign Relations, United States Senate*, 3 November 1981 (Washington, DC: US Government Printing Office, 1981), p. 44.

47. US Arms Control and Disarmament Agency, *Arms Control and Disarmament Agreements, Texts and Histories of Negotiations* (Washington, DC, US Government Printing Office, 1982), p. 52.

48. Max Lerner, *The Age of Overkill* (New York: Simon and Schuster, 1962), pp. 42-44.

49. N.C. Livingstone and J.D. Douglas, Jr., *CBW: The Poor Man's Atomic Bomb* (Cambridge: Institute for Foreign Policy Analysis, February 1984), National Security Paper # 1.

50. Jonathan Schell, *The Abolition* (New York: Alfred A. Knopf, 1984).

51. Herman Kahn, *On Thermonuclear War*, pp. 376-377.

52. Julian Perry Robinson, *Chemical Weapons and Chemical Arms Control*, edited by Matthew Messelson (New York: Carnegie Endowment for International Peace, 1977), p. 24.

53. N.C. Livingstone and J.D. Douglas, Jr., *CBW: The Poor Man's Atomic Bomb*, p. 7.

54. Ibid.

55. Ibid., p. 26.

206 NOTES TO CHAPTER 1

56. Julian Perry Robinson, *Chemical Weapons and Chemical Arms Control*, p. 24.

57. Committee of Soviet Scientists for Peace Against the Nuclear Threat, *Space-Strike Arms and International Security* (Moscow: October 1985), p. 49.

58. Albert L. Latter and Ernest A. Martinelli, *SDI: Defense or Retaliation* (Marina Del Rey: RDA/Logicon, 28 May 1985).

59. The letter to Dr. Albert Latter from Dr. Marvin C. Atkins, Deputy Director for Science and Technology, U.S. Defense Nuclear Agency, 7 August 1985, accompanies a list of comments. It makes it clear that the Latter and Martinelli paper is controversial. The letter begins, "to say that our people are skeptical is an understatement."

60. Gregory Canavan, "Countervalue Uses of Strategic Defense," Los Alamos National Laboratory Memorandum, P/AC:86-30, 2 May 1986.

61. Daniel Duedney, "Unlocking Space," *Foreign Policy*, Winter 1983-84, pp. 91-113.

62. Robert Heinlein, *The Moon Is a Harsh Mistress* (New York: Berkeley, 1984).

63. Stewart Nozette, editor, *Defense Applications of Near Earth Resources*, workshop held at the University of California, San Diego, Scripps Institute of Oceanography, 15-17 August, 1983 (La Jolla: California Space Institute, August 1983), Cal Space Ref. No. CSI83-3.

64. Giulio Douhet, *The Command of the Air*, p. 277.

65. Benson D. Adams, "Strategy and the First Strategic Defense Initiative," *Naval War College Review*.

66. Fletcher Pratt, *America and Total War* (New York: Smith and Durrell, Inc., 1941), p. 216.

67. Herman Kahn, *On Thermonuclear War*, p. 382.

68. General H.H. Arnold, "Third Report of the Commanding General of the Army Air Forces, 12 Nov 1945," in *The War Reports* (J.B. Lippincott Company, 1974), p. 464.

69. Bernard Brodie, in *The Absolute Weapon*, edited by Bernard Brodie (New York: Harcourt, Brace and Co., 1946).

70. Robert S. McNamara, *Statement of the Secretary of Defense before the House Armed Services Committee*, 30 January 1963, Department of Defense, p. 46.

71. Robert S. McNamara, *Statement by Secretary of Defense Robert S. McNamara on the Fiscal Year 1969-73 Defense Program and the 1969 Defense Budget*, Feb. 1968, Department of Defense, p. 42.

72. Glenn Kent, *A Summary Study of Strategic Offensive and Defensive Forces of the U.S. and USSR* (Washington, DC: The Director of Defense Research and Engineering, 8 Sept, 1964), p. 146.

73. Robert S. McNamara, *The Essence of Security: Reflections in Office* (New York: Harper and Row, 1969), pp. 63-64.

74. Robert S. McNamara and Hans A. Bethe, *Atlantic Monthly,* July 1985, p. 45.

75. Bernard Brodie, in *The Ultimate Weapon,* p. 59.

76. The text of the debate between Richard Garwin and Simon Worden was published by The United States Space Foundation, *Space Expectations* (Colorado Springs: US Space Foundation, 1986), pp. 159-179. The articles surveyed for emotional appeals were: (Pro-SDI:) Edward Teller, *Commentary,* March 1985, p. 4, Lowell Wood, *Commentary,* March 1985, p. 6, Robert Jastrow, *Commentary,* March 1985, pp. 17-22, Gerold Yonas, *Physics Today,* June 1985, pp. 34-31; and Edward Teller, *Discover,* September, 1985, pp. 66-75. Anti-SDI were: Carl Sagan, *Discover,* September, 1985, pp. 66-75, Wolfgang K.H. Panofsky, *Physics Today,* June 1985, pp. 33-45, Hans A. Bethe, Richard L. Garwin, Kurt Gottfried, Henry W. Kendall, Carl Sagan, and Victor F. Weisskopf, *Commentary,* March 1985, pp. 6-11; and Ashton B. Carter, *Commentary,* March 1985, pp. 11-12.

77. Hans A. Bethe, *et al., Commentary,* March 1985, p. 10.

78. Union of Concerned Scientists, *Space-Based Missile Defense* (Cambridge: Union of Concerned Scientists, March 1984), p. 32.

79. Testimony of Richard L. Garwin before the Senate Committee on Armed Services, 98th Congress, Second Session, 24 April 1984 (Washington, DC: US Government Printing Office, 1984).

80. Hans Bethe, Richard Garwin, Kurt Gottfried and Henry Kendall, "Space-Based Ballistic Missile Defense," *Scientific American,* October 1984, pp. 39-49.

81. After publication of the Union of Concerned Scientists March 1984 report and Ashton B. Carter, "Directed Energy Missile Defense in Space," US Congress, Office of Technology Assessment, Background Paper OTA-BP-ISC-26, April 1984, the Department of Defense asked the Lawrence Livermore and Los Alamos National Laboratories to prepare analyses on laser weapons constellation sizes. These reports (Gregory Canavan, *et al.,* "Comments on the OTA Report on Directed Energy Missile Defense in Space," Los Alamos National Laboratory, Report LA-UR-85-3572, May 1984 and C.T. Cunningham, Report No. DDV-84-007, Lawrence Livermore National Laboratory, 30 August 1984) endorsed previous Department of

Defense assessments that the correct number of laser satellites for the problem originally posed by the Union of Concerned Scientists was about 100.

82. The mathematical development of this argument is reviewed by Gregory Canavan and A. Petschek, "Satellite Allocation for Boost Phase Missile Intercept," Los Alamos National Laboratory, LA-UR-86-3245, 1986. Dr. Petschek has been a critic of SDI policy, having previously written a paper along with another SDI critic, A. Petschek and H. Bethe, "Scaling of Defensive Laser Satellite Constellations in 'Star Wars'," Los Alamos National Laboratory Report, LA-UR-85-2675, August 1985.

83. Richard Garwin and Simon Worden engaged in numerous public debates at universities throughout the United States between 1984-85. The laser constellation sizing issue always came up. Garwin published an essentially correct analysis in "How Many Orbiting Lasers for Boost-Phase Intercept?," *Nature,* 23 May 1985, pp. 286-290. In these calculations he adds parameters not present in the March 1984 Union of Concerned Scientists publication that he co-authored, i.e., new types of offensive missiles and new types of missile basing. With these additions he was able to derive laser constellation sizes larger than the original Department of Defense numbers. In the Colorado Springs debate (see note 76), he showed these constellation calculations and asserted that no one knows the correct answer to the laser constellation problem. This is of course sleight of hand. There are very specific answers for specific problems.

84. Study on Eliminating the Threat Posed by Nuclear Ballistic Missiles, James C. Fletcher, Study Chairman, *Volume VII, Soviet Countermeasures and Tactics,* Alexander H. Flax, Panel Chairman (Washington, DC: Institute for Defense Analyses, October 1983).

85. In Richard Garwin, "Space Weapons," *Bulletin of the Atomic Scientists,* May 1981, pp. 48-53, he calculated that 70 laser satellites would be able to destroy 400 ICBMs. These lasers are of lower performance than those postulated by Garwin in the 1984-85 debate. However, correcting for the differences in laser power and using the equations Garwin gives in his 1985 *Nature* article, I derive the number of about 80-90 lasers for the problem posed in the March 1984 Union of Concerned Scientists report. Note that Garwin co-authored the latter report, which contradicted the published number of 2400 lasers.

86. Richard Garwin waged a letter writing campaign against his critics on the laser constellation sizing issue. These letters were directed at senior officials in the National Laboratories where Garwin's critics

worked and to senior leadership within the Department of Defense. Garwin complained about my behavior in the latter letters. The content of these letters is reviewed in "IBM Scientist Complains about Opponents," *Military Space,* September 16, 1985, pp. 1, 4-6.

87. The statement that "MAD is a fact of life" occurs in essentially those words in articles by those critical of non-MAD strategies. For example, see Michael MacGuire, "Deterrence: The Problem, Not the Solution," *SAIS Review,* Summer-Fall 1985, pp. 105-124, and Spurgeon Kenny, Jr. and Wolfgang K.H. Panofsky, "MAD vs. NUTS: Can Doctrine or Weaponry Remedy the Mutual Hostage Relationship of the Superpowers?" *Foreign Affairs,* Winter 1981/82, pp. 387-404.

88. Comments made by Albert Wohlstetter at the Defense Nuclear Agency New Alternatives Workshop, 25 June 1986, Falls Church, Virginia.

89. Montgomery C. Meigs, *Managing Uncertainty: Vannevar Bush, James B. Conant and the Development of the Atomic Bomb, 1940-45,* Ph.D. Thesis, University of Wisconsin-Madison, 1982, pp. 184-221.

90. Albert Einstein, *Out of My Later Years* (New York: Philosophical Library, 1950), p. 138.

91. For a review of Albert Einstein's political efforts in support of world government see Paul Doty, "Einstein and International Security," in *Albert Einstein: Historical and Cultural Perspectives,* edited by G.H. Molton and Y. Elkona (Princeton: Princeton University Press, 1982), pp. 347-368.

92. Bertrand Russell reviewed the origins of Pugwash and dealings with Albert Einstein in his book, *Has Man a Future?* (New York: Simon and Schuster, 1962), pp. 47-67. I am personally skeptical of the Pugwash Conferences' political approach based on an incident in 1985 where I was invited and later "disinvited" by the US conference organizers due to objections from other US participants that I was an overzealous supporter of the SDI. No such strictures are placed on Soviet participants, who are expected to zealously support their government's positions.

93. Bertrand Russell, *Common Sense and Nuclear Warfare* (New York: Simon and Schuster, 1959), p. 88.

94. Ibid., pp. 36-38.

95. Robert Jervis, in *Deterrence Theory Revisited,* Center for Arms Control and International Security, University of California, Los Angeles, Working Paper #14, April 1979, identifies three stages in deterrence theory evolution. The first was Brodie's 1940s work and

similar ideas. The second was the late 1950s and early 1960s work by analysts such as Herman Kahn and Henry Kissinger. The third "wave," which considers deterrence as part of the problem as much as the solution, can be found in Glen H. Snyder and Paul Diesing, *Conflict Among Nations* (Princeton: Princeton University Press, 1977) and Alexander L. George and Richard Smoke, *Deterrence in American Foreign Policy: Theory and Practice* (New York: Columbia University Press, 1974).

96. An excellent review of the Catholic bishops' 1983 pastoral letter, *The Challenge of Peace: God's Promise and Our Response,* and the development of deterrence and morality arguments within the Catholic traditions of "Just War" and "Pacifism" is provided by James E. Dougherty, *The Bishops and Nuclear Weapons* (Cambridge: Archon Books, 1984).

97. After the Catholic bishops' review of the morality of deterrence, several Protestant groups took a more radical approach and rejected deterrence more firmly. In 1986 the United Methodist Council of Bishops released *In Defense of Creation: The Nuclear Crisis and a Just Peace* (Nashville: Graded Press, 1986).

98. See, for example, Jonathan Schell, *The Abolition* (New York: Alfred A. Knopf, 1984) and Freeman Dyson, *Weapons and Hope* (New York: Harper and Row, 1984).

2. Retaliation-Based Nuclear Deterrence

1. Karl von Clausewitz, *On War* (Princeton: Princeton University Press, 1976).

2. Ibid., p. 77.

3. Ibid., p. 78.

4. Soviet preoccupation with Clausewitz is well known. Lenin's annotated copy is an icon of special sanctity to the Soviets. It is curious that the Soviets deified an imperialist general who worked for the Russian Tsar. What appealed to Lenin, and presumably still does to Soviet

ideologues, is Clausewitz's central premise that war is policy and politics. One of the best discussions of Soviet ideology and Clausewitz is given by Byron Dexter, "Clausewitz and Soviet Strategy," *Foreign Affairs*, October 1950, pp. 41-51.

5. I hasten to note that Secretary of State Dulles's famous Massive Retaliation speech in 1954 (*Department of State Bulletin*, 25 January 1954) did not say that cities or the enemy population were our nuclear target.

6. Henry Kissinger, *Nuclear Weapons and Foreign Policy* (New York: Harper and Brothers, 1957).

7. Maxwell D. Taylor, *The Uncertain Trumpet* (New York: Harper and Brothers, 1959). Other Flexible Response advocates who had significant impact were William W. Kaufmann, editor and author, *Military Policy and National Security* (Princeton: Princeton University Press, 1956) and Robert E. Osgood, *Limited War: The Challenge to American Security* (Chicago: The University of Chicago Press, 1957).

8. Secretary of Defense Robert McNamara (1961-1968) originally identified two strategic missions—Damage Limiting and Assured Destruction. The latter prevented war, the former operated if deterrence failed. McNamara's book, *Blundering Into Disaster* (New York: Pantheon, 1986) charts the evolution of his thinking as Secretary of Defense. Damage Limitation progressively receded in importance.

9. The Nixon administration firmly rejected MAD and returned its rhetoric to a "warfighting" basis. For an authoritative review of Nixon Administration strategy see his Defense Secretary Melvin Laird's article, "A Strong Start in a Difficult Decade: Defense Policy in the Nixon-Ford Years," *International Security*, Fall 1985, pp. 5-26.

10. President Carter's "countervailing" strategy was formulated in Presidential Directive (PD) 59. His Secretary of Defense, Harold Brown, reviewed PD-59 in a speech at the Naval War College, 20 August 1980. See "Excerpts From Address on War Policy," *New York Times*, 21 August 1980, p. A-9.

11. Henry A. Trofimenko, "Counterforce: Illusion of a Panacea," *International Security*, Spring 1981, pp. 28-48.

12. General David Jones, Hearings before the Committee on Armed Services, United States Senate, Ninety-Sixth Congress, First Session, 24 June 1979 (Washington: U.S. Government Printing Office, 1979), pp. 169-170. The quote was from General Jones' response to a question on MAD by Senator John Tower.

13. J.F.C. Fuller, *The Conduct of War, 1786-1961* (New Brunswick: Rutgers University Press, 1961), p. 286. Major General Fuller was

regarded by many as the father of flexible response. At the end of World War II he wrote of the need for limited war options in his book *Armament and History* (New York: Scribners, 1945).

14. Paul Kosemchak, unpublished manuscript, Research and Development Associates, Inc., Arlington, VA, 1986.

15. Fuller, *The Conduct of War*, p. 302.

16. Henry S. Rowen, "The Evolution of Strategic Nuclear Doctrine," in *Strategic Thought in the Nuclear Age*, Laurence Martin, editor (Baltimore: Johns Hopkins University Press, 1979), p. 137.

17. Samuel F. Wells, Jr., "The Origins of Massive Retaliation," *Political Science Quarterly*, Spring 1981, pp. 22-52.

18. For a review of the debates among the nuclear bomb-builders, see Daniel J. Keyles, *The Physicist* (New York: Knopf, 1977).

19. Edward Teller, letter in *Commentary*, March 1985, p. 4. Teller cites Andrei Sakharov, father of the Soviet hydrogen bomb, to the effect that the Soviet H-bomb effort was well under way years before the public US debate over the weapon's feasibility and desirability.

20. A.J. Bacevich, *The Pentomic Era: The U.S. Army Between Korea and Vietnam* (Washington, DC: National Defense University Press, 1986).

21. Maxwell D. Taylor, *The Uncertain Trumpet*. General Taylor returned from retirement to serve as Chairman of the Joint Chiefs of Staff in the Kennedy administration.

22. Ibid., p. 6.

23. Ibid., p. 146.

24. Ibid., p. 116.

25. John Foster Dulles, *Foreign Affairs*, October 1957.

26. Maxwell D. Taylor, *The Uncertain Trumpet*, p. 171.

27. Ibid., p. 76.

28. James M. Gavin, *War and Peace in the Space Age* (New York: Harper and Brothers, 1978).

29. Ibid., p. 248.

30. There were many important strategic analyses in the late 1950s— the "Golden Age" of nuclear strategy. I believe the following cover the waterfront on "Flexible Response":

    a. Paul H. Nitze, "Atoms, Strategy, and Policy," *Foreign Affairs*, January 1956, pp. 187-198.

    b. Henry Kissinger, "Force and Diplomacy in the Nuclear Age," *Foreign Affairs*, April 1956, pp. 349-366.

c. Albert Wohlstetter, "The Delicate Balance of Terror," *Foreign Affairs*, January 1959, pp. 211-234.

31. Paul H. Nitze, "Atoms, Strategy and Policy," *Foreign Affairs*, January 1956, p. 187.

32. Henry Kissinger, *Nuclear Weapons and Foreign Policy*. This book expands on the premises of Dr. Kissinger's 1956 *Foreign Affairs* article.

33. Ibid., p. 132.

34. Albert Wohlstetter, "The Delicate Balance of Terror." *Foreign Affairs*, January 1959, pp. 211-234.

35. Robert McNamara, "The United States and Western Europe: Concrete Problems of Maintaining a Free Community," *Vital Speeches*, 1 August 1962, p. 628.

36. Morton H. Halperin, *Defense Strategies for the Seventies* (Boston: Little, Brown and Company, 1971), p. 74.

37. Richard M. Nixon, *U.S. Foreign Policy for the 1970s* (Washington, DC: U.S. Government Printing Office, 1970), p. 122.

38. James R. Schlesinger, *Annual Defense Department Report* (Washington, DC: U.S. Government Printing Office, 1974), pp. 25-45. See particularly p. 39.

39. Henry S. Rowen, "The Evolution of Strategic Nuclear Doctrine."

40. Colin S. Gray, "Nuclear Strategy: The Case for a Theory of Victory," *International Security*, Summer 1979, pp. 54-87. A shorter version of Gray's ideas appeared in 1980. Colin S. Gray and Keith Payne, "Victory Is Possible," *Foreign Policy*, Summer 1980, pp. 14-27.

41. Colin S. Gray, "Nuclear Strategy," p. 56.

42. Harold Brown's remarks at the Naval War College, 20 August 1980.

43. For a thorough review of "countervailing strategy," see an article written by senior Carter administration official Walter Slocombe, "The Countervailing Strategy," *International Security*, Spring 1981, pp. 18-27.

44. Fred C. Iklé, "Can Nuclear Deterrence Last Out the Century?" *Foreign Affairs*, January 1973, pp. 267-285.

45. Ibid., p. 272. For readers not familiar with MAD's moral antecedents, Tomas de Torquemada (1420-1489) was a Dominican friar who served as the first Grand Inquisitor for the Spanish Inquisition. In 1478 Pope Sixtus IV granted a bull authorizing the Catholic rulers of Spain

to establish an inquisition, called the "Tribunal of the Holy Office," that would eliminate nominally baptized Jews and Moslems suspected of secret recidivism. That meant virtually all of them. As Grand Inquisitor, Friar Tomas's name became synonymous with the extreme cruelty of the measures used to extract confessions. From Robert Held, *Inquisition* (Florence: Qua D'Arno, 1985).

46. Paul H. Nitze, "Assuring Strategic Stability in an Era of Detente," *Foreign Affairs*, January 1976, pp. 207-232. Nitze's efforts and his longstanding reputation as a strategic thinker and arms control expert were instrumental in generating opposition to the Salt II Treaty within the US Senate in 1979.

47. Ibid., p. 206.

48. This division is attributed to General Glenn Kent, McNamara's strategic expert. I have been unable to find a paper within which Kent laid out this formulation. However, during a strategic stability conference held 21-23 October 1986 at the Naval War College most speakers attributed these ideas on stability to him. General Kent, who was present, was quick to remind those who forgot that he had originated the idea.

49. Richard Lee Walker, *Strategic Target Planning: Bridging the Gap Between Theory and Practice* (Washington, DC: National Defense University Press, 1983), p. 14.

50. Paul H. Nitze, "Deterring Our Deterrent," *Foreign Policy*, Winter 1976-1977, pp. 195-210.

51. The first quantitative treatment of static measures and their application to arms control was Glenn Kent, "On the Interaction of Opposing Forces Under Possible Arms Control Agreements," Occasional Papers in International Affairs, #5, March 1963, Center for International Affairs, Harvard University. Since assured destruction was the stated basis for deterrence at the time, Kent considered those measures most relevant to assured destruction, for example total megatonnage.

52. Henry Kissinger, *Nuclear Weapons and Foreign Policy*, p. 74.

53. Paul H. Nitze, "Deterring Our Deterrent," *Foreign Policy*, Winter 1976-77, p. 200.

54. Edward L. Warner III, Glenn A. Kent, Randall J. Devalk, "Key Issues for the Strategic Offensive Portion of the Nuclear and Space Talks in Geneva," *RAND Note N-2348-1-AF* (Santa Monica: RAND Corporation, December 1985), p. iv.

55. Ibid., p. 12.

56. Paul H. Nitze, "Deterring Our Deterrent," *Foreign Policy*, Winter 1976-77, p. 200.

57. For discussions on the growing number of Chinese, British and French warheads and their growing warfighting potential see Christopher Campbell, *Nuclear Weapons Fact Book* (Novato, CA: Presidio, 1984) and *Nuclear Weapons Proliferation and Nuclear Risk*, ed. James A. Shear (New York: St. Martin's Press, 1984).

58. Unclassified data from a briefing given to the SDI Organization by the Organization of the Joint Chiefs of Staff/J-5.

59. For example, Richard Lee Walker's *Strategic Target Planning* (Washington, DC: National Defense University Press, 1983).

60. See, for example, Paul H. Nitze, "Deterring Our Deterrent," p. 200.

61. Karl von Clausewitz, *On War*, pp. 119-121.

62. I participated in two JCS wargames in 1985. Both games explored potential US and Soviet moves and countermoves associated with US deployment of space-based strategic defenses. All games included senior advisors and officials. These are the people who would make the decisions in real crises.

63. Much of the information in this section comes from studies done by senior strategists for the Rockwell Corporation and the Office of the Secretary of Defense. The data cited come from unclassified portions of a briefing by M.I. Yarymovich and F.X. Kane, *Meeting Our Strategic Objectives in the 1990s* (El Segundo: Rockwell International Corporation, 86-190-S, 8 April 1986).

64. Walker, *Strategic Target Planning*.

65. Nitze, "Assuring Strategic Stability in an Era of Detente."

66. M.I. Yarymovich and F.X. Kane, *Meeting Our Strategic Objectives in the 1990s,* Chart RI-4-86039.

67. Robert S. McNamara, *Statement of Secretary of Defense Before the House Armed Services Committee. The Fiscal Year 1965-69 Defense Program and 1965 Defense Budget*, 27 January 1964, pp. 31-32.

68. Colin S. Gray and Keith Payne, "Victory Is Possible," *Foreign Policy*, Summer 1980, pp. 14-27.

69. *Soviet Military Power*, 1987, p. 52.

70. M.I. Yarymovich and F.X. Kane, *Meeting Our Strategic Objectives in the 1990s*, Chart RI-4-86039.

71. From a letter written to Cardinal Bernardin, 15 January 1983, by National Security Advisor William Clark. Cited in James E. Dougherty, *The Bishops and Nuclear Weapons* (Cambridge: Archon Books, 1984).

72. J.F.C. Fuller, *The Conduct of War 1786-1961*, p. 264.

73. Colin S. Gray, "Nuclear Strategy," p. 66, discusses US economic targeting. He cites General Brown's quote as support of his discussion. The quote originally appeared in *The Defense Monitor*, Vol. VI, No.6, August 1977, p. 2.

74. *Soviet Military Power*, 1987, pp. 45-61.

75. These numbers are consistent with many sources. See for example *Soviet Military Power*, 1987, pp. 41-57. The effectiveness of Soviet defenses is very difficult to estimate. I assume that Soviet defenses have significant capability based on the fact that *Soviet Military Power*, 1987, specifically discusses the topic, stating "The Soviets have probably violated the [ABM Treaty] provisions on testing surface-to-air missile (SAM) components in an ABM mode by conducting tests involving the use of SAM air defense radars in ABM-related testing activities. Moreover, the SA-10 and SA-X-12 SAM systems may have the potential to intercept some types of strategic ballistic missiles."

76. M.I. Yarymovich and F.X. Kane, *Meeting Our Strategic Objectives in the 1990s*, Chart RI-4-86038.

77. Harold Brown, "Is SDI Technically Feasible?" *Foreign Affairs*, Vol. 64, Fall/Winter 1985-86, pp. 435-454.

78. Robert S. McNamara, *Blundering Into Disaster*, pp. 89-91.

79. Interview with Robert S. McNamara, 8 December 1986. Mr. McNamara referred to ideas on how to handle a transition to a defense-reliant deterrent—namely President Reagan's cooperative transition proposal made to Soviet General Secretary Gorbachev at the October 1986 Iceland summit—as "crap. " He felt strongly enough about this to repeat the metaphor twice.

80. Karl von Clausewitz, *On War*, p. 84.

81. Ibid., p. 357.

82. Ibid., pp. 357-365.

83. Robert S. McNamara, *Blundering Into Disaster*, p. 98.

84. *Star Wars: Delusions and Dangers* (Moscow: Military Publishing House, 1985), p. 31.

85. *Soviet Military Power*, 1987, pp. 45-61.

86. Glenn A. Kent and Randall J. DeValk, *Strategic Defenses and the Transition to Assured Survival* (Santa Monica: RAND Corporation, R3369-AF, 1986).

87. C. Max, P. Banks, M. Cornwall, F. Dyson, S. Flatte, O. Rothaws, J. Sullivan and F. Zachariasen, *Deployment Stability of Stratgic Defenses* (McLean: JASON/MITRE, JSR 85-926, October 1986).

3. Non-Nuclear Deterrence

1. Sun Tzu, *The Art of War* (London: Oxford University Press, 1971), pp. 77-78.

2. Karl von Clausewitz, *On War* (Princeton: Princeton University Press, 1984), pp. 90-91.

3. Bernard Brodie, *The Absolute Weapon* (New York: Harcourt Brace and Co., 1946), pp. 76-77.

4. This is a key excerpt from President Reagan's 23 March 1983 speech, a speech later labeled as "Star Wars" by Senator Edward Kennedy of Massachusetts. This title was quickly adopted for Reagan's concept by SDI critics. The complete text of the speech is given in "A Decision Which Offers a New Hope for Our Children," *Washington Post*, 24 March 1983, p. A12.

5. What deters war is the burning question of the nuclear age. Surprisingly, deterrent theorists seldom turn to history for lessons. One of the few historical investigations of deterrence is R. Narroll, V.L. Bullough, and F. Naroll, *Military Deterrence in History: A Pilot Cross-Historical Survey* (New York: SUNY Press, 1974). The survey covers 120 periods of history for nine different civilizations during the past 2000 years. It attempts to correlate the type of strategy (offensive or defensive), military strength, geographical, diplomatic, cultural, and administrative situations with the workings of deterrence. Surprisingly, almost nothing other than strong cultural connections with a potential adversary led to stable deterrence.

6. Sun Tzu, *The Art of War*, p. 114.

7. Ibid., p. 85.

8. Interview with former Secretary of Defense Robert S. McNamara, Washington, DC, 8 December 1986.

9. General of the Army H.H. Arnold, "Third Report of the Commanding General of the Army Air Forces," in *The War Reports*, edited by Walter Millis (New York: J.B. Lippincott Company, 1947).

10. Ibid.

11. Bernard Brodie, *The Absolute Weapon*, pp. 25-30, discusses, and dismisses, statements by Admiral Nimitz and President Truman (*New York Times*, 6 Oct 1945, p. 6) that less than perfect defenses against the atomic bomb are both feasible and desirable. Traditional defense experts, such as J.F.C. Fuller, *Armament and History* (New York: Scribners, 1945), p. 194, also expressed optimism that the atomic bomb could be used to defend even better than it could be used for an attack.

12. Bernard Brodie, *The Absolute Weapon*, p. 30.

13. Edward R. Jayne II, *The ABM Debate* (Cambridge, MA: Massachusetts Institute of Technology, Center for International Studies, Ph.D. Dissertation, June 1969).

14. David N. Swartz, "Past and Present: The Historical Legacy," in *Ballistic Missile Defense*, edited by Ashton B. Carter and David N. Swartz (Washington, DC: The Brookings Institution, 1984) pp. 330-349.

15. Henry Kissinger, *Nuclear Weapons and Foreign Policy* (New York: Harper and Brothers, 1957), p. 411, cited efforts in 1950 by a group of Massachusetts Institute of Technology scientists to emphasize a defense-oriented strategy. Kissinger also noted the fervent opposition of airpower advocates to this approach.

16. Cited in *Aviation Week*, Volume 59, November 23, 1953, pp. 16-17.

17. Edward R. Jayne II, *The ABM Debate*, p. 40, cites a 1957 RAND study sponsored by the Air Force which rejected population defense in favor of defending only deterrent forces. Excerpts from this study appeared in *Aviation Week*, Volume 67, 14 October 1957, p. 37.

18. These criticisms were contained in the 1957 RAND report cited in note 17.

19. David M. Swartz, *Ballistic Missile Defense*, p. 332.

20. Advocates of strategic defense in the late 1950s, losing in the Pentagon, took their case to Congress. This was the first direct interest Congress took in ballistic missile defense with an eye toward modifying the Administration's strategic posture. Although the House Armed

Services Committee under Carl Vinson eventually endorsed the Eisenhower Pentagon approach, the proceedings make interesting reading and are contained in *Investigations of National Defense Missiles*, Committee on Armed Forces, US House of Representatives, 85th Congress, 2nd Session, January-February 1958 (Washington, DC: US Government Printing Office, 1958).

21. The fact that he established ARPA as a missile defense initiative in the State of the Union message shows President Eisenhower's recognition of the intense public and Congressional interest in this subject. The text of the message can be found in *New York Times*, January 10, 1957.

22. Edward R. Jayne II, *The ABM Debate*, pp. 105-113.

23. Ibid., p. 175.

24. Ibid., p. 176.

25. Ibid., p. 222.

26. Glenn Kent, *A Summary Study of Strategic Offensive and Defensive Forces of the US and USSR* (Washington, DC: The Director of Defense Research and Engineering, Department of Defense, 8 September 1964).

27. Edward R. Jayne II, *The ABM Debate*, p. 144.

28. The Atmospheric Test Ban has prevented the United States from getting data similar to that obtained by the Soviets. One of the key arguments used by critics of strategic defenses has been that they will not work in a nuclear environment. The critics also point out that we can never get realistic data on these effects—a fact they have assured through arms control. Only the Soviet Union has real data on this question.

29. *Pravda*, 23 February 1965.

30. Edward R. Jayne II, *The ABM Debate*, p. 185.

31. Ibid., p. 186.

32. Sayre Stevens, "The Soviet ABM Program," in *Ballistic Missile Defense*, edited by Ashton B. Carter and David N. Swartz (Washington, DC: The Brookings Institution, 1984), pp. 192-197.

33. Ibid., p. 198.

34. Ibid., p. 205.

35. Sayre Stevens, *Ballistic Missile Defense*, p. 357.

36. Robert S. McNamara, *Blundering into Disaster* (New York: Pantheon Books, 1986), p. 57.

37. Edward R. Jayne II, *The ABM Debate*, p. 368.

38. The text of Secretary McNamara's San Francisco speech is given in *U.S. News and World Report*, 2 October 1967, pp. 106-111.

39. The text of President Nixon's 14 March 1969 speech is given in *Safeguard: Why the ABM Makes Sense*, edited by Willian Kintner (New York: Hawthorn Books, 1969), pp. 1-7.

40. D.G. Brennan, "The Case for Population Defense," in *Sageguard: Why the ABM Makes Sense*, pp. 207-241.

41. Books by opponents of the Safeguard ABM and defense-reliant strategies were readily available in paperback and widely touted by the liberal press. In the 1969 debate the principal critics' book, *ABM: An Evaluation of the Decision to Deploy an Anti-Ballistic Missile System*, edited by Abram Chayes and Jerome Wiesner (New York: Signet Books, 1969) was on the streets in paperback in May 1969—only two months after President Nixon's speech announcing Safeguard deployment. Books by proponents, such as the one cited in notes 39 and 40, appeared only in hardback a year or more later.

42. Abram Chayes, Jerome B. Wiesner, George W. Rathjens, and Steven Weinberg, in *ABM: An Evaluation of the Decision to Deploy an Anti-Ballistic Missile System*, p. 24.

43. Ibid., p. 27.

44. Ibid., p. 44. When I visited Beijing in June 1987, Chinese government officials told me that they didn't fear the SDI because they could develop countermeasures. Under questioning, it was clear that they had no specifics in mind, but were repeating the arguments of the 1960s ABM critics.

45. Ibid., p. 36.

46. Ibid., pp. 41-42.

47. Bernard T. Feld, "The ABM and Arms Control," in *ABM: An Evaluation of the Decision to Deploy an Anti-Ballistic Missile System*, pp. 187-192.

48. "An Introduction," in *ABM: An Evaluation*, pp. 17-24.

49. A most damaging and egregious article against the 1969 ABM deployment decision was by Richard L. Garwin and Hans Bethe, "Anti-Ballistic Missile Systems," *Scientific American*, March 1968, pp. 21-31. This article was widely touted in 1969 as "proof" of the infeasibility of ABM. Its principal objection to Safeguard was the "blackout" problem, whereby a high-altitude nuclear burst would mask follow-on nuclear warheads from the ABM radar. This article was misleading on a number of grounds. See, for example, the

discussion by D.G. Brennan cited in note 54. Richard L. Garwin was also at the forefront of the 1980s anti-SDI debate. During the latter period he also widely disseminated data that was shown to be technically erroneous. See notes 78-85 to chapter 1.

50. Jerome B. Wiesner, "Some First-Strike Scenarios," in *ABM: An Evaluation*, p. 79.

51. Leonard S. Rodberg, "ABM Reliability," in *ABM: An Evaluation*, pp. 107-117, and J.C.R. Licklider, "Overestimates and Overexpectations," in *ABM: An Evaluation*, pp. 118-129. These articles made statements such as, "Many engineers feel that it will simply not be possible to program such a [ABM] computer successfully in the near future." Safeguard was built a few years later and the truth about the computers was much different, as cited by N.H. Brown, M.P. Fabisch, and C.J. Rifenberg, the Safeguard systems engineers in *The Bell System Technical Journal*, 1975. They wrote, "It can reasonably be said that the complete development, including the integration of the first installed sites, was performed on schedule and that the system met the prescribed specifications."

52. Albert Wohlstetter, "The Delicate Balance of Terror," *Foreign Affairs*, January 1959, pp. 211-234.

53. See Melvin R. Laird, Secretary of Defense Testimony in Hearings before Subcommittees of the Committee on Appropriations, House of Representatives, 91st Congress, First Session, 22 May 1969 (Washington, DC: US Government Printing Office, 1969), pp. 5-39.

54. For a discussion of this particular piece of disinformation see D.G. Brennan, "The Case for Population Defense," in *Safeguard: Why the ABM Makes Sense*, p. 214.

55. Sayre Stevens, in *Ballistic Missile Defense*, p. 202.

56. Ibid., p. 204.

57. The history of the SALT I negotiations and the commitment of the arms controllers to using these negotiations as a means to further MAD strategy is documented by John Newhouse, *Cold Dawn: The Story of SALT* (New York: Holt, Rinehart and Winston, 1973).

58. Hearings on the Military Implications of the Treaty on the Limitation of Antiballistic Missile Systems and the Interim Agreement on Limitation of Strategic Offensive Arms before the Senate Armed Services Committee, 20 June 1972 (Washington, DC: US Government Printing Office, 1972), p. 383.

59. Ibid., p. 111.

60. Ibid., p. 186, testimony of D.G. Brennan.

61. Ibid., pp. 219-225, testimony of Edward Teller.

62. The Senate Armed Services Committee hearings on the ABM Treaty were dominated by the late Senator Henry Jackson's unsympathetic questions. This contrasted with the friendly reception received by Treaty advocates in the Senate Foreign Relations Committee hearings going on at the same time. Senator Henry ("Scoop") Jackson played one of the most important roles in assuring a strong national defense. He was the last of the "old time" pro-defense liberals. Clearly on the left on social issues, he also pushed hard for a strong US strategic posture. His efforts often resulted in effective bipartisan support for strategic initiatives. His presence was surely missed in the 1980s. The liberal wing of the Democratic party has come to uniformly condemn the SDI and any other move that smacks of strategic competition. It is almost as if, to be a liberal, one must attempt to believe that there are no external threats to the United States. "Scoop" Jackson's legacy extended into the 1980s through his former adviser, Richard Perle, who, as Assistant Secretary of Defense for International Security Policy in the Reagan administration, continued the tradition of a strong defense going hand in hand with a "liberal intellectual" approach.

63. The US Unilateral Statement A to the ABM Treaty was made on 9 May 1972, only weeks before the Treaty was submitted for ratification. The full text of this statement is in *Arms Control and Disarmament Agreements* (Washington, DC: US Government Printing Office, Arms Control and Disarmament Agency, 1982), p. 146. The late date of this statement suggests that it was a response to demands by Senator Henry Jackson, among others, to link defensive limits to offensive limitations. For a discussion of this issue see John Newhouse, *Cold Dawn*, pp. 200-202.

64. See testimony by John Foster, Director of Defense Research and Engineering, before the Senate Armed Services Committee, 20 June 1972, p. 222.

65. *Arms Control and Disarmament Agreements*, pp. 161-163.

66. John Newhouse, *Cold Dawn*, pp. 230-231. In 1971, after much interagency controversy, it was decided that the United States would seek to ban all activities related to mobile "exotic" ABM systems such as lasers. In 1985 the Reagan administration decided that the United States had failed to convince the Soviets to agree to this ban. This reinterpretation of the ABM Treaty became a major political fight in 1986 and 1987, and is still the subject of an intense public debate.

67. Based on my review of the 1972 ABM Treaty negotiating record.

68. Abraham Sofaer, Legal Advisor to the Department of State, *The ABM Treaty, Part I: Treaty Language and Negotiating History*

(Washington, DC: Office of the Legal Advisor, Department of State, 11 May 1987).

69. *Pravda*, September 30, 1972.

70. The Union of Concerned Scientists, *Empty Promise: The Growing Case Against Star Wars*, edited by John Tirman (Boston: Beacon Press, 1986), pp. 203-204. The ABM Treaty is cited as the basis for "the arms control regime that has served U.S. security interests admirably."

71. Following the Defensive Technologies and Future Security Strategies Studies of the summer of 1983, National Security Decision Directive (NSDD) 119 was issued in January 1984. It established the Strategic Defense Initiative (SDI). A summary of the two study results is in *Defense Against Ballistic Missiles: An Assessment of Technologies and Policy Implications* (Washington, DC: US Government Printing Office, April 1984).

72. Articles addressing the technical futility and strategic undesirability of defense-reliant deterrence were frequent prior to President Reagan's March 1983 speech. For example, Richard Garwin published a 1981 attack on the feasibility of laser-based defenses in "Are We on the Verge of a New Arms Race in Space?" *Bulletin of the Atomic Scientists*, May 1981, pp. 48-55. See also Spurgeon Keeney, Jr., and Wolfgang K.H. Panofsky, "MAD vs. NUTS: The Mutual Hostage Relationship of the Superpowers," *Foreign Affairs*, Winter 1981/82, pp. 287-304.

73. Richard Pipes, "Why the Soviet Union Thinks It Could Fight and Win a Nuclear War," *Commentary*, September 1977, pp. 21-34. See also Richard Pipes, "Team B: The Reality Behind the Myth," *Commentary*, October 1986, pp. 25-40.

74. The Committee on the Present Danger was founded in 1976 by a bipartisan group of prominent defense figures. Among these were Paul Nitze, Eugene V. Rostow, Dean Rusk, Lane Kirkland, Max Kampelman, Richard Allen, David Packard, and Henry H. Fowler. Team B included Richard Pipes, Lt. Gen. John Vogt, Major General Jaspar Welch, Jr., Paul Nitze, Lt. Gen. Daniel O. Graham, Professor William van Cleave, Foy Kohler, Paul Wolfowitz, Thomas Wolfe and Seymour Weiss. Nitze became President Reagan's Arms Control Advisor, Kampelman his chief strategic negotiator, and Richard Allen his first National Security Advisor. Richard Pipes served for a time as the Soviet specialist in Reagan's National Security Council staff.

75. Most notable of these studies was the 1982 Defense Science Board study chaired by former Defense Research and Engineering Director John Foster.

76. General Graham's High Frontier systems studies were first published in 1982 and republished in early 1983. They were entitled *High Frontier: A Strategy for National Survival* (Washington, DC: High Frontier, 1982).

77. For a discussion of these space-laser proposals and Senator Wallop's support for them, see "ABM Promise Seen in Space-Based Laser," *Aviation Week*, 8 October 1979, p. 15, and Clarence A. Robinson, Jr., "Space-Based Laser Battle Stations Seen," *Aviation Week*, 8 December 1980, p. 36.

78. The SDI's scientific critics invariably attribute the concept to Edward Teller. See, for example, the Union of Concerned Scientists, *Empty Promise*, p. 3. Although Dr. Teller did brief his nuclear X-ray concept to President Reagan, it did not become a favored idea. The Defensive Technologies Study, or "Fletcher" Study, team did not include any X-ray laser experts, nor did it include Teller on its advisory group. As a member of this team, I was well aware of the acrimonious debate over the exclusion of X-ray laser proponents. This exclusion was deliberate. The public report of the Fletcher Study, *The Strategic Defense Initiative: Defensive Technologies Study* (Washington, DC: US Government Printing Office, April 1984) made no mention of Teller's X-ray laser concept.

79. The Joint Chiefs of Staff met with President Reagan on 11 February 1983 (see "Reagan for the Defense," *Time*, 4 April 1983, p. 11). The following information is based on my discussions with James C. Fletcher, Director of the Defensive Technologies Study, and with Dr. George Keyworth, science advisor to the President. The Chiefs of Staff initiated discussions of the SDI and were enthusiastic supporters. During a briefing of the Defensive Technologies Study by Fletcher to them in September 1983, it was clear to me that they had played a major role in starting the Strategic Defense Initiative.

80. The Keyworth studies reportedly identified ground-based lasers as the most promising missile defense approach. See Boyce Ransberger, "White House Science Advisor is a Cheerleader for Reagan," *Washington Post*, November 12, 1985, p. A6.

81. William Broad, " 'Star Wars' Traced to Eisenhower Era," *New York Times*, October 28, 1986, p. C1.

82. The first public discussion of the feasibility of a near-term space-based missile defense by a Reagan administration official was my 1986 paper entitled "What Can We Do? When Can We Do It?" *National Review*, December 31, 1986, pp. 36-40.

83. This survivability argument has figured prominently in every critical article on the SDI. It was, in fact, quickly recognized by the

Fletcher Study team in 1983 that space system survivability was a critical issue. However, the team also recognized that there are many promising approaches to solving the problem.

84. Data from the Office of the Assistant Deputy Chief of Staff for Space Systems, USAF, January 1987.

85. Secretary of Defense Caspar Weinberger, Pentagon News Conference, cited in *Star Wars Quotes* (Washington, DC: Arms Control Association, July 1986), p. 4.

86. Presidential Science Advisor George A. Keyworth III, in an address to aerospace contractors, May 21, 1985, cited in *Star Wars Quotes*, p. 5.

87. Admiral James Watkins, "Keeping *Teeth* in the Policy of Deterrence," *Defense 85*, March 1985, pp. 14-18.

88. Keith Payne, *Star Wars in Perspective* (Lanham, MD: Hamilton Press, 1986), pp. 233-247.

89. *Star Wars Quotes*, p. 99.

90. Ibid.

91. European concern resulted in numerous meetings between European leaders and President Reagan. The most significant of these was between British Prime Minister Margaret Thatcher and President Reagan at Camp David in early 1985. Mrs. Thatcher agreed to support the SDI under four conditions: Western objectives must not include strategic superiority; BMD deployment is to be negotiated with the Soviets; deterrence must be enhanced; and negotiations with the Soviets must focus on offensive reductions. For a discussion of allied reactions, see Keith Payne, *Strategic Defense*, Chapter 10.

92. The Soviets always translate US and Western references to deterrence into Russian as "Ustrasheniye," which means "frightening" or "intimidating." On the other hand the Soviets have a concept of deterrence which they consistently express with the Russian word "Zderzhivaniye," which means "restraint" or "holding back." The latter comes much closer to the purpose of defense-reliant deterrence. I thus identify "Ustraheniye" as punishment deterrence, and "Zderzhivaniye" as denial deterrence. See Phillip A. Peterson and John G. Hines, "The Conventional Offensive in Soviet Theater Strategy," *Orbis*, Vol. 27, No. 3, Fall 1983, pp. 695-739.

93. The threatening nature of Soviet translations of the English word "deterrence" underlies several proposals for changing our basic strategy. See, for example, Freeman Dyson, *Weapons and Hope* (New York: Harper and Row, 1984).

94. It's difficult to find unclassified information on warhead reliability. The only data I can find is of 1960s vintage in Daniel Fink, "Strategic Warfare," *Science and Technology*, October 1968, p. 54. He estimates ICBM reliability at between 41 and 65 percent.

95. Arms Control Association, *Star Wars Quotes*.

96. *The President's Strategic Defense Initiative* (Washington, DC: US Government Printing Office, January 1969).

97. Address by Ambassador Paul Nitze, Special Advisor to the President and Secretary of State for Arms Reduction Negotiations before the World Affairs Council of Philadelphia, 20 February 1985. The speech is published in *The Strategic Defense Debate: Can 'Star Wars' Make Us Safe?* (Philadelphia: The University of Pennsylvania Press, 1986), pp. 221-227.

98. National Security Decision Directive (NSDD) 172. The substance of this directive is published in US State Department Special Report No. 129, "The Strategic Defense Initiative," June 1985.

99. The Union of Concerned Scientists, *Empty Promise*, p. 11.

100. After months of delay, the June 1986 (originally due in March 1986) *Report to Congress on the Strategic Defense Initiative* (Washington, DC: Department of Defense, June 1986) stated cost-effectiveness in these convoluted terms:

> Third, we will consider, in our evaluation of options generated by SDI research, the degree to which certain types of defensive systems, by their nature, encourage an adversary to overwhelm them with additional offensive capability while other systems can discourage such a counter effort. We seek defensive options — as with other military systems — that are able to maintain capability more easily than countermeasures could be taken to defeat them. This criterion is couched in terms of cost-effectiveness. However, it is much more than an economic concept.

101. Among "countermeasures" to SDI, the Soviets usually place attacks on satellite components first. See, for example, *Weaponry in Space: The Dilemma of Security* (Moscow: MIR Publishers, 1986).

102. Robert S. McNamara, "The Military Role of Nuclear Weapons: Perceptions and Misperceptions," *Foreign Affairs*, Fall 1983, pp. 59-80.

103. Glenn A. Kent, "Sensible Goals for Star Wars," *Washington Post*, 4 January 1987, p. C2.

104. Quoted by J.F.C. Fuller, *Armament and History*, p. 87.

105. For a discussion of ancient Greek military ethics see James E. Dougherty, *The Bishops and Nuclear Weapons* (Cambridge, MA: Archon Books, 1984), pp. 36-37.

106. Ibid., pp. 40-43.

107. J.F.C. Fuller, *Armament and History*, p. 37.

108. I spent more than a year on the US strategic arms delegation in Geneva from 1985-86. I was surprised to find the Soviets presenting small personal gifts—books with photos of churches, small art objects, items for one's wife, etc. Such "humanizing" gifts made it more difficult to press the US case in a hardnosed manner.

109. Freeman Dyson, *Weapons and Hope*. Jonathan Schell, *The Fate of the Earth* (New York: Alfred A. Knopf, 1982). Jonathan Schell, *The Abolition* (New York: Alfred A. Knopf, 1984). The U.S. Catholic Bishops' Pastoral Letter, *The Challenge of Peace: God's Promise and Our Response*, 1983.

110. Each of the works cited in Note 109 condemns warfighting strategies in even stronger terms than MAD.

111. Quoted by James E. Dougherty, *The Bishops and Nuclear Weapons*, p. 146. Contained in the Bishops' Pastoral Letter, p. 15.

112. The United Methodist Council of Bishops, *In Defense of Creation: The Nuclear Crisis and Just Peace* (Nashville: Graded Press, 1986).

4. Disarmament: A Non-Deterrent Strategy

1. Sun Tzu, *The Art of War* (London: Oxford University Press, 1971), p. 100.

2. Comment made by Winston Churchill on the signing of the Soviet-Nazi non-aggression pact in 1939. This event surprised and shocked the world, since the two signatories had diametrically opposed political systems.

3. I served on the US delegation to the nuclear and space arms talks with the Soviet Union from March 1985 until May 1986. During this period the Soviet Union continued its unabated aggression in Afghanistan, a US Army major in East Germany was murdered, and a nuclear plant in Chernobyl blew up (and the Soviets lied about it for weeks). They also turned the US Space Shuttle *Challenger* disaster into an opportunity to decry "US militarization of space." None of these actions were consistent with stated Soviet goals of lowered tension.

4. Prior to the November 1985 summit the Soviets handed out a typewritten diatribe against SDI by the Committee of Soviet Scientists for Peace, Against the Nuclear Threat, *Space Strike Arms and International Security* (Moscow: October 1985). The Soviets have also produced and distributed two glossy attacks on the SDI. They were widely distributed in the United States and heralded by the liberal press. One, also by the Committee of Soviet Scientists, is *Weaponry in Space: The Dilemma of Security* (Moscow: Mir Publishers, 1986), and the other is *'Star Wars': Delusions and Dangers* (Moscow: Military Publishing House, 1985). The Soviet Scientists for Peace are often those working hardest on the Soviet missile defense and military space efforts. See *The Soviet Propaganda Campaign Against the Strategic Defense Initiative* (Washington, DC: US Government Printing Office, Arms Control and Disarmament Agency, August 1986).

5. I attended several conferences on SDI in Western Europe between 1985 and 1987. Three of these, two in West Germany and one in Great Britain, had representatives from Georgi Arbatov's USA/Canada Institute. During a meeting sponsored by the Aspen Institute/Berlin, General Bogdanov of the KGB typified Soviet approaches by sporting a 1960s-vintage Western peace emblem. The image of a KGB general adorned with a peace symbol is not to be forgotten. The 1986 Pugwash meeting in Great Britain had four USA/Canada representatives, but the organizers had disinvited all official US representatives because of their alleged "bias" toward the Administration position.

6. Quoted by Raymond L. Garthoff, *Soviet Military Doctrine* (Glencoe, IL: The Free Press, 1953), p. 13.

7. Karl von Clausewitz, *On War* (Princeton: Princeton University Press, 1984), p. 69.

8. Quoted by Raymond L. Garthoff, *Soviet Military Doctrine*, p. 55. Lenin was fascinated by Clausewitz. His copy of *On War* is annotated in his own hand and is a Soviet national treasure on display in Moscow. The statement given here was written in August 1915 and was published in Lenin's *Socialism and War*, 1933.

NOTES TO CHAPTER 4   229

9. Karl von Clausewitz, *On War*, p. 370.

10. From Lenin's commentary on Clausewitz, cited by Garthoff, p. 11.

11. In 1917, the young Soviet Russian Republic badly needed peace with the Germans so it could turn its attention to countering internal opposition to Bolshevik rule. It signed the Brest-Litovsk Treaty with the Germans, ceding large amounts of Russian-claimed territory to Germany. The "one step back—two steps forward" statement was Lenin's response to critics of this seeming surrender.

12. Alexis de Tocqueville, *Democracy in America*, Bradley and Phillips, eds. (New York: Knopf, 1944).

13. Richard Pipes, *Russia Under the Old Regime* (New York: Charles Scribner's Sons, 1974).

14. Ibid., pp. 3-5.

15. Ibid., p. 78.

16. See, for example, Marshal V.D. Sokolovskiy, *Soviet Military Strategy*, 3rd Edition, translated by Harriet Fast Scott (New York: Crane, Russek and Co., 1968). This seminal 1960s book on Soviet strategy was originally published in 1968 (Moscow: Voyenizdat, 1968). Earlier editions appeared in 1962 and 1963.

17. Richard Pipes, *Russia Under the Old Regime*, pp. 115-120.

18. Since M.S. Gorbachev became General Secretary in March 1985, numerous Western commentators have praised the "momentous" changes he has brought about. This policy of "Glasnost" or "openness" may or may not be in the West's interest. I prefer the pessimistic view that Gorbachev follows the ideology of his hard-line sponsors, such as the late Stalinist ideologue Mikhail Suslov, and is following the classic Soviet "one step back, two steps forward" approach. An excellent summary of this pessimistic assessment is Michael W. Johnson, "Gorbachev's Detente—The KGB Connection," *Military Intelligence*, Vol. 12, No. 4, October-December 1986, pp. 6-11.

19. See Richard Pipes' discussion of Peter the Great in *Russia Under the Old Regime*, pp. 113-128.

20. Raymond L. Garthoff, *Soviet Military Doctrine*, p. 49.

21. Ibid., p. 4.

22. Ibid., p. 18.

23. Both Garthoff's 1953 review of Soviet World War II strategy and Sokolovskiy's 1960s summary stress the Soviet "scientific" approach and Soviet condemnation of "adventurist" Western strategy.

24. Raymond L. Garthoff, *Soviet Military Doctrine*, p. 82.

25. Ibid., p. 52.

26. V.D. Sokolovskiy, *Soviet Military Strategy*, p. 135.

27. Garthoff, p. 174.

28. Sokolovskiy, p. 159.

29. Garthoff, p. 302.

30. Ibid., p. 326. Garthoff cites Soviet World War II aviation expert Colonel N. Denisov on the subordinate role of aviation to ground forces in "The Offensive Power of Soviet Aviation," *Krasnaia Zvezda*, 16 and 17 August 1944.

31. Ibid., p. 151. Garthoff cites Soviet 1930s military expert L.S. Anuragov, "On the Military Theoretical Heritage of Marx-Engels-Lenin," *Voina i Revoluitsica*, No. 1, January-February, 1934, p. 64.

32. Henry Kissinger, *Nuclear Weapons and Foreign Policy* (New York: Harper and Brothers, 1957), p. 388.

33. Garthoff, p. 175, cites Marshal of Aviation Vershinin, *Pravda*, 17 July 1949, in rejecting single-weapon strategies such as the air power theories of Douhet.

34. Henry Kissinger, *Nuclear Weapons and Foreign Policy*, p. 365.

35. John G. Hines, Phillip A. Peterson, and Notra Trulock III, "Soviet Military Theory for 1945-2000: Implications for NATO," *The Washington Quarterly*, Fall 1986, pp. 83-89.

36. Marshal V.D. Sokolovskiy's *Soviet Military Strategy* appeared in three editions. The best translation, which identifies the additions and deletions from edition to edition, is the one by Harriet Fast Scott cited in Note 16.

37. Ibid., p. 190.

38. Ibid., p. 230.

39. Ibid., p. 275.

40. Ibid., p. 291.

41. Ibid., p. 255.

42. Ibid., p. 280. The preemptive doctrine was explicit only in the Third Edition, 1968.

43. Hines, *et al.*, "Soviet Military Theory," cite recent Soviet criticisms of Sokolovskiy for its reliance on massive ICBM strikes. Most notable of these criticisms is a 1985 book by the Soviets' chief military scientist, Colonel General M.A. Gareyev, *M.V. Frunze—Military Theoretician: The Views of M.V. Frunze and Contemporary Military Theory* (Moscow: Voyenizdat, 1985).

44. Edward R. Jayne II, *The ABM Debate* (Cambridge, MA: Massachusetts Institute of Technology, Center for International Studies, Ph.D. dissertation, June 1969), p. 368.

45. Ambassador Gerard Smith, testimony in Hearings before the Senate Armed Services Committee on Military Implications of the Treaty on the Limitation of Antiballistic Missile Systems and the Interim Agreement of Limitations of Strategic Offensive Arms, 20 June 1972 (Washington, DC: US Government Printing Office, 1972), p. 383. Ambassador Smith was asked by Senator Henry Jackson if he believed that the Soviets accepted MAD. Smith replied, "I think that the Soviets, as a result of the SALT negotiations, have moved toward accepting the concept of assured destruction."

46. During my 1985-86 tenure as an advisor to the US delegation to the negotiations on nuclear and space arms with the Soviet Union, the US team frequently cited 1960s Soviet writings as evidence of Soviet interest in warfighting and the role of strategic defense. One of the Soviet negotiators gave me a book by the Soviet Deputy Foreign Minister, V. Petrovskiy, *Security in the Nuclear Space Area* (Moscow: International Relations Publishing House, November 1985). The Soviets said they were tired of US references to old strategy and wanted us to be aware of their current thinking. The quote given here appears in the DIA Translation, LN-670-86, 19 August 1986, p. 65.

47. Stephen M. Meyer, "Soviet Strategic Programs and the US SDI," *Survival*, November-December 1985, pp. 274-292. Meyer cites these assured destruction numbers from K.V. Tarakanov, *Mathematica i Voorzhenneva bor'ba* (Moscow: Voyenizdat, 1974), pp. 184-186.

48. The key correlation of forces equations for nuclear weapons were set forth in 1967, at the height of Soviet reliance on nuclear-armed ICBMs, by Major General I. Anureyev, "Determining the Correlation of Forces in Terms of Nuclear Weapons," *Voyennaya Mysl (Military Thought*—the classified Soviet General Staff journal), No. 6, 1967.

49. The sophisticated Soviet Correlation of Forces modeling in terms of nuclear weapons is more complex than Anureyev's paper provides. See David Geske, *Operational Decision Making in Soviet Military Affairs* (Arlington, VA: SRS Technologies, February 1986).

50. US Military Posture Statement for FY 1985 prepared by the Organization of the Joint Chiefs of Staff, given in hearings before the Committee on Armed Services, US Senate, 98th Congress, 2nd Session, 1 February 1984 (Washington, DC: US Government Printing Office, 1984). Page 123 gives ratios of total US and Soviet megatonnage. Page 435 provides these ratios in more militarily meaningful equivalent megatonnage, or EMT. See also figure 5.

51. For a summary of these Correlation of Forces results see Stephen M. Meyer in *Survival*, November-December 1985, p. 284.

52. *Soviet Strategic Defense* (Washington, DC: US Government Printing Office, October 1985).

53. *Soviet Military Power* (Washington, DC: US Government Printing Office, 6th Edition, March 1987), p. 45.

54. Michael J. Deane, *Strategic Defense in Soviet Strategy* (Washington, DC: Advanced International Studies Institute, 1980), p. 22.

55. Freeman Dyson, *Weapons and Hope*.

56. *The Strategic Defense Initiative*, Department of State Special Report No. 129, June 1985, p. 3. This report contains the policy mandated in National Security Decision Directive (NSDD) 172.

57. V.D. Sokolovskiy, *Soviet Military Strategy*, p. 283.

58. Ibid., p. 13.

59. *Star Wars: Delusions and Dangers*, p. 31.

60. See Note 11.

61. Soviet emphasis on retreat as a form of offensive was discussed by Raymond L. Garthoff, *Soviet Military Doctrine*, Chapter 10, pp. 157-163.

62. Raymond L. Garthoff, *Soviet Military Doctrine*, p. 356.

63. Michael J. Deane, *Strategic Defense in Soviet Strategy*, p. 24.

64. Marshal of the Soviet Union R. Ya. Malinovskiy, Minister of Defense, speech, in XXII CPSU Congress, Volume II (Moscow: Politizdat, 1962), p. 117.

65. For a discussion of the development, deployment, and capabilities of 1960s Soviet missile defense systems, see Michael J. Deane, *Strategic Defense in Soviet Strategy*, Chapter 3, pp. 23-45; Sayre Stevens, "The Soviet BMD Program," in *Ballistic Missile Defense*, edited by Ashton B. Carter and David N. Schwartz (Washington, DC: The Brookings Institution, 1984), pp. 182-220; and Carnes Lord, "Taking Soviet Defenses Seriously," *The Washington Quarterly*, Fall 1986, pp. 101-116.

66. Sayre Stevens, "The Soviet BMD Program," p. 192.

67. Michael J. Deane, *Strategic Defense in Soviet Strategy*, p. 36.

68. N. Talenskiy, "Anti Missile Systems and the Problems of Disarmament," *Mezhdunarodnaya Zhizn (International Affairs)*, no. 10, October 1964, pp. 28-34. Reprinted in *The Bulletin of the Atomic*

Scientists, February 1965, pp. 25-29. The appearance of General Talenskiy's article in a left-leaning Western disarmament journal and his attendance at Pugwash conferences suggest that his article may have been designed more for Western audiences than as an indication of Soviet thinking. See Carnes Lord, "Taking Soviet Defenses Seriously," (Note 65) for a discussion of this issue.

69. Ibid., *Bulletin of the Atomic Scientists* translation.

70. See, for example, the introduction to the Soviet anti-SDI publication, *Weaponry in Space: The Dilemma of Security*, pp. 11-16. It cites a number of Western anti-SDI articles. Throughout this and other Soviet publications specific numbers and technical ideas are always cited as being from "Western sources." This furthers the charade that the Soviets do not have an SDI-type program. For more discussion of this issue, see *The Soviet Propaganda Campaign Against the US Strategic Defense Initiative*, a US Government publication, cited in Note 4.

71. Michael J. Deane, *Strategic Defense in Soviet Strategy*, pp. 55-65.

72. See *Soviet Strategic Defense Programs*, (Washington, DC: US Govenment Printing Office, October 1985) for a discussion of Soviet missile defense programs since 1972.

73. Soviet Minister of Defense Andrei A. Grechko, *Pravda*, 30 September 1972.

74. Michael J. Deane, *Strategic Defense in Soviet Strategy*, pp. 95-98.

75. Marshal of Aviation G.V. Zimin, *Development of Anti-air Defense* (Moscow: Voyenizdat, 1976), p. 192. Cited by Carnes Lord, "Taking Soviet Defenses Seriously," p. 89.

76. Carnes Lord, "Taking Soviet Defenses Seriously," p. 84.

77. V.D. Sokolovskiy, *Soviet Military Strategy*, p. 255.

78. N. Talenskiy, "Anti Missile Systems."

79. N.V. Ogarkov, *Always Ready to Defend the Motherland* (Moscow: Voyenizdat, 1982), p. 36. Cited by Carnes Lord, "Soviet Defense," pp. 84-85.

80. Gorbachev's "Glasnost" bears striking resemblance to the years immediately following Stalin's death, when Khrushchev made new overtures to the West. Some were not fooled. See, for example, Dennis Healey, "When Shrimps Learn to Whistle," *International Affairs*, Vol. 32, 1956, pp. 1-10. Khrushchev's quote, from which Healey took his article's title, is contained in remarks to East German journalists on 17 September 1955.

81. Cited by V. Petrovskiy, *Security in the Nuclear Space Area*, p. 87.

82. For an excellent discussion of Soviet "peace" offensives prior to World War II, see T.A. Taracouzio, *War and Peace in Soviet Diplomacy* (New York: Macmillan, 1940). Lenin's 1917 "Peace Decree" is discussed on page 57.

83. See, for example, Garthoff, *Soviet Military Doctrine*, pp. 256-257.

84. V.D. Sokolovskiy, *Soviet Military Strategy*, p. 15.

85. V. Petrovskiy, *Security in the Nuclear Space Area*, p. 50.

86. Ibid.

87. Ibid., p. 6.

88. Ibid., p. 51.

89. Ibid., p. 145.

90. Ibid., p. 48.

91. Ibid., pp. 66 and 96.

92. Ibid., cited on p. 64.

93. Sokolovskiy's first edition carried much discussion on the promise of space for Soviet military use. These discussions were deleted in later editions. The incorrect Kennedy quote is given on page 456 of Harriet Fast Scott's translation. The correct President Kennedy quote was, "Control of space will be decided in the next decade, and the nation which controls space can control the Earth," in *Missiles and Rockets*, 24 October 1960, p. 13.

94. The 1967 Outer Space Treaty may go down in history as the worst such endeavor ever undertaken by the United States. It contains absolutely no provisions for verification and was purely the result of "arms control for arms control's sake." For a discussion of the events leading up to its creation and a text, see *Arms Control and Disarmament Agreements* (Washington, DC: US Government Printing Office, 1982), pp. 48-58.

95. *Soviet Military Space Doctrine* (Washington, DC: US Government Printing Office, 1 August 1984), p. 21.

96. Ibid., p. 28.

97. During the 1985 nuclear and space talks in Geneva the Soviet delegation insisted for six months that a multimegawatt laser at Sary Shagan was a "medical" laser. The Soviet publication, *Weaponry in Space*, cited in note 4, quotes Soviet Defense Minister Marshal Sokolov: "The USSR does not work in this area [space-based ballistic missile defense]," p. 110.

98. National Security Council unclassified memorandum, dated 18 October 1986, entitled, "Reykjavik Chronology." This was the only summary of what transpired during the October 1986 summit meeting between President Reagan and General Secretary Gorbachev.

99. V. Petrovskiy, *Security in the Nuclear Space Area*, p. 2.

100. Committee of Soviet Scientists, *Space Strike Arms and International Security (Abridged)*, p. 49. See also Note 4.

Conclusion: US Strategic Defense

1. For a discussion of the primary role military weakness played in the fall of the Western Roman Empire, see Arthur Ferrill, *The Fall of the Roman Empire: The Military Explanation* (London: Thames and Hudson, 1986).

2. The solution of the Republican party and conservative strategists to US national security problems is to make better use of US technological strengths. Contrasted with the Democrats, Republicans favor technological fixes. Republican support of the SDI derives in part from this view. See, for example, Daniel O. Graham, *High Frontier: Strategy for National Survival* (Washington, DC: High Frontier/TOR Books, 1983).

3. In the twilight years of the Roman Empire there were at least some who were concerned and who proposed imaginative solutions to the Empire's problems. Among the best known is an illustrated proposal for some exotic war machines to stem the barbarian tide—*De Rebus Bellicus*. Unfortunately, the author's name is unknown. A translation and commentary on this work is provided by E.A. Thompson, *A Roman Reformer and Inventer* (Oxford: Clarendon Press, 1952).

4. Current US debate on how to redress the weakening of US military power relative to our adversaries is fierce. The Democratic party, and liberals in general, counsel renewed emphasis on basic military skills. See, for example, Gary Hart and William S. Lind, *America Can Win: The Case for Military Reform* (Bethesda, MD: Adler & Adler, 1986).

5. A traditionalist view on how to save the Roman empire was provided by a military man, Flavius Vegettius Renatus. His *De Re Militari* proposed a return to rigorous military training. A text is

supplied by Major Thomas R. Phillips, *Roots of Strategy* (Harrisburg: Telegraph Press, 1940), pp. 65-175.

6. Report of the President's Commission on Strategic Forces (Scowcroft Commission) (Washington: US Government Printing Office, 1983).

7. Public comments in 1987 by senior Department of Defense strategists such as Richard Perle, Assistant Secretary of Defense for International Security Policy, and Fred Iklé, Under Secretary of Defense for Policy, increasingly opposed the proposed Midgetman single-warhead ICBM.

8. In late 1986 the Union of Concerned Scientists gave the Midgetman its "partial" support. This was the only strategic system so supported.

9. The Soviet SA-12B "Giant" missile is an anti-tactical ballistic missile (ATBM). It has been fully field tested against intermediate-range missiles. A warhead without sophisticated penetration aids—such as an SLBM or a single-warhead Midgetman—may well be vulnerable to the SA-12B. For more details, see *Soviet Military Power* (Washington, DC: US Government Printing Office, March 1987), pp. 49-50.

10. It would cost $200 million for a 10-warhead MX, according to figures given by the Congressional Office of Technology Assessment in *MX Missile Basing* (Washington: US Government Printing Office, OTA-ISC-140, September 1981). This cost includes missile, warhead, and silo-basing. Mobile systems are considerably more expensive.

11. The 1983 Scowcroft Commission (see Note 6) cautioned against early US deployment of strategic defenses. It feared triggering a near-term Soviet response. Information obtained from Senator Malcolm Wallop's office shows that, in mid-1986, when President Reagan was confronted with demands by conservative Republican senators for near-term missile defense deployments, he responded that the Joint Chiefs of Staff objected to such deployments. They had done so, he said, on the grounds that Soviet defenses could be more rapidly deployed. These arguments were published by Willian F. Buckley in the *Washington Post*. Mr. Buckley's information reportedly came directly from the President.

12. The "many decades away" view on missile defense deployments is the liberal, MAD view. See a staff report written for two liberal Democratic senators by Douglas C. Waller and James T. Bruce, *SDI: Progress and Challenges, Part Two*, Staff Report Submitted to Senator William Proxmire and Senator J. Bennett Johnson, 19 March 1987. Warfighting advocates are more positive about deployments, but

are still skeptical that they could be deployed in the next decade. See Paul Nitze, "An Arms Control Agenda that Kissinger Should Know," *Washington Post*, 30 March 1987, Section A, p. 11. Nitze was responding to Kissinger's urging for immediate deployments of missile defenses.

13. A number of articles and papers by qualified scientists and engineers appeared in late 1986 pointing out the possibilities for near-term defensive deployments. Among these are my own "What Can We Do? When Can We Do It?" *National Review*, 31 December 1986, pp. 36-40, and The George C. Marshall Institute, *Missile Defense in the 1990s* (Washington, DC: George C. Marshall Institute, 1987).

14. Department of Defense, *Soviet Military Power*, p. 47.

15. Ibid., p. 48.

16. V. D. Sokolovskiy, *Soviet Military Strategy, 3rd Edition*, translated by Harriet Fast Scott (New York: Crane Russak and Company, 1980), contrasts Soviet counterforce targeting (p. 275) with aggressive "imperialist" countervalue targeting (p. 277).

17. The SDI Organization submits an annual description of technologies and systems to Congress. As of this writing, the most recent is *Report to Congress on the Strategic Defense Initiative* (Washington, DC: Department of Defense, April 1987).

18. George C. Marshall Institute, *Missile Defense in the 1990s*, p. 10.

19. William J. Broad, "Star Wars Traced to Eisenhower Era," *New York Times*, 28 October 1986, Section C, p. 1. This article provides a short history of missile defense work in the United States.

20. For example, the 1969 anti-ABM book, *ABM: An Evaluation of the Decision to Deploy an Antiballistic Missile System*, edited by Abram Chayes and Jerome Wiesner (New York: Signet, 1969) had several articles about computer programming: Leonard S. Rodberg, "ABM Reliability," pp. 107-117, and J.C.R. Licklider, "Overestimates and Over Expectations," pp. 118-129. These articles rejected the possibility of constructing reliable Safeguard software.

21. The Safeguard software was completed on schedule, within costs, and meeting specifications. N.H. Brown, M.P. Fabisch, and C.J. Refenberg, "Safeguard Data Processing System: Introduction and Overview," *Bell System Technical Journal*, 1975, pp. S9-S25.

22. The Union of Concerned Scientists, *Empty Promise: The Growing Case Against Star Wars*, edited by John Tirman (Boston: Beacon Press, 1986), article by Greg Nelson and David Redall, "Could We Trust the SDI Software?" pp. 87-106.

23. Soviet Scientists Committee for the Defense of Peace Against Nuclear Threat, *Weaponry in Space: The Dilemma of Security* (Moscow: Mir, 1986), p. 92.

24. *Study on Eliminating the Threat Posed by Nuclear Ballistic Missiles*, James C. Fletcher, Study Chairman, Volume VI, Battle Management, Brock Adams, Panel Chairman (Washington, DC: Institute for Defense Analyses, 1983).

25. Statement by Solomon J. Buchsbaum, AT&T Bell Laboratories, 3 December 1985, before the United States Senate Committee on Armed Services, Subcommittee on Strategic and Theater Nuclear Forces (Washington, DC: US Government Printing Office, 1985).

26. James C. Fletcher, "The Technologies for Ballistic Missile Defense," *Issues in Science and Technology*, Vol. I, pp. 15-29.

27. In early 1985 the SDI Organization responded to criticism on the feasibility of effective software for a global defense system by commissioning several studies. These studies concluded that no exotic methods, such as "artificial intelligence," were needed—just intelligent application of existing software technologies. The studies were submitted as follows:

Eastport Study Group Summer Study 1985, "A Report to the Director, Strategic Defense Initiative Organization," December 1985.

Report on the Workshop for Automated Software Programming, Alvin M. Despain, Chairman (McLean, VA: JASON/Mitre Corporation, JSR-85-927, February 1986).

For a summary of these results, see M. Mitchell Waldrop, *Science*, 9 May 1986, pp. 710-713.

28. George C. Marshall Institute, *Missile Defense in the 1990s*, pp. 12-17.

29. Ibid., p. 7.

30. SDI proponents' data set an initial defense, more robust than my System A, at 93 percent effective and costing $121 billion (George C. Marshall Institute, *Missile Defense in the 1990s*, p. 8). In Senate testimony, Lt. General James A. Abrahamson, SDI Director, placed the initial system effectiveness at about 40 percent with a cost of between $40-60 billion. Individual component costs put forward by SDI critics, for example Barry M. Blechman and Victor Utgoff, *Fiscal and Economic Implications of Strategic Defense* (Baltimore: Johns Hopkins Foreign Policy Institute, 23 July 1986), use component costs similar to mine but differ markedly in the total number of components required. The main difference between advocate and critic cost

estimates is not in the unit costs, but in the level of countermeasures of the Soviets and in the assumption of how effective the system must be.

31. The Space Shuttle Orbiter weighs about 105 kilograms and costs $3 billion to replace (data from NASA Headquarters). The NASA Space Telescope weighs about 104 kilograms and would cost about $500 million to replicate (data from NASA Headquarters). The Defense Meteorological Satellite weighs about 103 kilograms and costs about $30 million per copy (data from the principal contractor, RCA Astroelectronics, Princeton, NJ).

32. The 1983 Defensive Technologies Study concluded that the Soviets could not introduce new types of offensive systems, such as fast-burn boosters, into their inventory until after the year 2000.

33. George C. Marshall Institute, *Missile Defense in the 1990s*, pp. 40-41. A fake ICBM capable of fooling the sophisticated missile defense sensors would cost 90 percent of the cost of a real ICBM.

34. George C. Marshall Institute, *Missile Defense in the 1990s*, pp. 9-10 is the source for EXO GBI (called the Exo-Atmospheric Reentry Vehicle Intercept System, or ERIS, in this report) data. The study team was fully briefed on these systems by the SDI Organization.

35. Most of the public debate in 1984-1985 centered on exotic, space-based laser systems. These long-term defensive possibilities were the focus of Congressional, scientific and Soviet attacks on the SDI. Examples:

Ashton B. Carter, *Directed Energy Missile Defense in Space—A Background Paper* (Washington, DC: US Congress, Office of Technology Assessment, OTA-SP-ISC-16, April 1984).

The Union of Concerned Scientists, John Tirman, editor, *The Fallacy of Star Wars* (New York: Random House, 1985).

Committee of Soviet Scientists for Peace, Against the Nuclear Threat, *Space-Strike Arms and International Security* (Moscow: October 1985).

36. The fast-burn booster is the favorite countermeasure of SDI critic Richard Garwin, "The Soviet Response: New Missiles and Countermeasures," in *Empty Promise*, pp. 129-146.

37. See Note 33.

38. Richard Garwin, "The Soviet Response," in *Empty Promise*, p. 131.

39. Ibid., p. 132.

40. Data from the US Air Force Office of ICBM Modernization. Richard Garwin, in ''The Soviet Response,'' *Empty Promise*, p. 133, claims these are ''goldplated'' numbers.

41. One of the most interesting SDI debates of the mid-1980s had nothing to do with strategy, but dealt with an analytical question of how many space-laser battle stations would be needed to counter a specified Soviet threat. The worst case, from the standpoint of the laser defense, is a large number of fast-burn boosters fired simultaneously from a small geographical area. The last word on this subject was published in a joint paper co-authored by an SDI proponent, G.H. Cananvan, and an SDI critic, A.G. Petschek, *Satellite Allocation for Boost-Phase Missile Intercepts* (Los Alamos, NM: Los Alamos National Laboratory, LA-10926-MS, April, 1987).

42. Data obtained from Richard Joseph, Special Assistant to the Director, SDI Organization, February 1987.

43. Many advocates of nuclear warfighting strategies prefer nuclear-armed ground-based interceptors. These systems can counter MaRVs and are most suitable for defending hard targets. Low-altitude defense missiles armed with nuclear weapons can damage or destroy the very soft targets they are designed to protect. See Sidney D. Drell, Phillip J. Farley, and David Holloway, *The Reagan Strategic Defense Initiative: A Technical, Political, and Arms Control Assessment* (Cambridge, MA: Ballinger, 1985).

44. The fact that future strategic defense system costs could fit easily within current strategic budgets, and not affect conventional force budgets, was discussed by Robert Cooper, ''A Moderate View,'' in *The Strategic Defense Debate: Can 'Star Wars' Make Us Safe?* edited by Craig Snyder (Philadelphia: The University of Pennsylvania Press, 1986), pp. 157-165.

45. The Soviets seem to prefer defense suppression as a counter-measure to space-based missile defenses. See Note 103, Chapter 3. The survivability of space systems always tops the list of US SDI critics. See John Tirman and Peter Didesheim, ''Lethal Paradox: The ASAT—SDI Link,'' in *Empty Promise*, pp. 107-128.

46. I do not believe that the current submarine deterrent situation will remain indefinitely stable. The Soviets are hard at work on means to detect and destroy Western submarines. Whether or not submarines are survivable is an interesting dilemma in the SDI debate. On the one hand, SDI critics say that US submarines are survivable and we don't need missile defenses to enhance an already stable deterrent. On the

other hand, SDI proponents point out that submarine survivability methods should be applicable to space systems. If SDI critics think subs are survivable, why don't they extend their analysis to satellites? For several exchanges on this topic, see United States Space Foundation, *Space Expectations* (Colorado Springs: US Space Foundation, 1986), pp. 176-179, and *Physics Today*, May 1987, p. 15.

47. Readers interested in the defense and vulnerability of World War I aircraft and the analogy with the current debate on satellite survivability will find interesting reading in F.W. Lanchester, *Aircraft in Warfare: The Dawn of the Fourth Arm* (London: Constable and Company, 1916).

48. US Congress, Office of Technology Assessment, *Ballistic Missile Defense Technologies* (Washington, DC: US Government Printing Office, OTA-ISC 254, September 1985).

49. See Note 45.

50. Department of Defense, *Soviet Military Power*, pp. 47-50.

51. Gregory Canavan, *An Assessment of Strategic Defenses* (Los Alamos NM: Los Alamos National Laboratory, 1987). Canavan specifically discusses satellite nuclear hardness possibilities.

52. John Tirman and Peter Didesheim, "The ASAT-SDI Link," in *Empty Promise*, p. 115.

53. The most serious threat against satellites is a ground-based laser. This threat has been the basis of Edward Teller's concern over space-based defensive systems (see *The Atlantic*, July 1985). A thorough review of this problem was done by Lowell Wood, "Concerning the Vulnerability of Objects in Space to Attack by Ground-Based Laser Systems" (Livermore, CA: Lawrence Livermore National Laboratory, 1986).

54. Although the application of air, sea, and space law to future strategic defense systems in space is an almost unexplored topic, there are some preliminary conclusions which I can draw on this subject.

> 1. Space law should follow precedents set by sea and air law. See George W. Ash, *1982 Convention on the Law of the Sea—Its Impact on Air Law* (London: University College LL.M. Thesis, 1 July 1985). For example, international treaty language dealing with mass destruction weapons on the seabed is similar to the sections dealing with the same weapons in outer space.

> 2. Recent naval and air engagements set a strong precedent for self-defense, even preemptive self-defense, when there are threats against free passage and survivability. For example, the United

States shot down Libyan jets in 1984 when those jets locked on missile guidance radar—prior to an actual attack. Israel destroyed an Iraqi nuclear plant in the late 1970s prior to a demonstrated nuclear capability by that country. In 1987, the United States warned Iran that it would destroy Chinese-supplied shore-to-ship missiles if any of those missiles were fired at US shipping.

I conclude that a ground-based laser attack on sovereign space assets would be met with vigorous countermeasures, including the destruction of that laser site, if necessary.

3. EPILOGUE

1. *Soviet Military Power, 1990*, Department of Defense, US Government Printing Office, S/N 008–000–00565–6, pp. 48–71.

2. In the fall of 1990, the SDI Organization restructured the SDI program toward "Protection Against Accidental Launch," with a specific focus against Third World threats. See "SDIO Shifts Focus, Prepares for Cuts," *Space News*, 8–14 Oct 1990, p. 1.

3. 8 March 1990, The White House, Statement by the Press Secretary on Space Policy.

4. Speech by Vice President Quayle before the American Institute of Aeronautics and Astronautics, 1 May 1990, Arlington, VA.

5. Japan appears to have targeted space as a major growth industry for the decades ahead. The Japanese Ministry of International Trade and Industry (MITI)—the key Japanese long-range planning agency—has begun encouraging Japanese industrial investment in space. The Moon and its potential uses are high on the Japanese agenda. Shimizu Corporation, the world's largest construction firm, has over 100 people working full time on space and lunar long-range planning (Shimizu Corporation pamphlet, *Up to Space*, 1989, Tokyo). In 1989 Japan launched the first probe to the Moon since the Soviet and US probes of the early 1970s. MITI has chartered studies into using space to supply energy to Earth. For more information, see "Asia in Space," *Space News*, pp. 6–13.

6. In 1989 NASA proposed an approach for responding to President Bush's commitment to return to the Moon and explore Mars: *Report of*

the 90 Day Study on Human Exploration of the Moon and Mars, November 1989, National Aeronautics and Space Administration. NASA identified seven critical technologies. In the 1990–91 "Synthesis" Study sponsored by NASA to further work out the proposed exploration program, the study team identified the SDI-developed technologies in three of the areas—advanced launch systems, nuclear-thermal propulsion, and space nuclear power—represented the most promising approaches.

7. Lowell Wood, "Concerning Advanced Architectures for Strategic Defense," Presented to the Strategic Defense Initiative: The First Five Years Conference, Washington, DC, 13–15 March 1988, Lawrence Livermore National Laboratory, UCRL–98434 Preprint. See also, Lowell Wood and Walter Scott, "Brilliant Pebbles," Presented at The Strategic Defense Initiative Technical Achievements Symposium, National Academy of Sciences, Washington, DC, 29–30 June, 1989. Lawrence Livermore National Laboratory, UCRL–101292 Preprint.

8. The author served as White House National Space Council staff officer for the Space Exploration Initiative (SEI) in 1989–90. The approach taken for the SEI—namely, to spend a few years on basic technology and alternate architecture development before starting on actual mission and system development—was deliberately modeled on the SDI.

9. US National Space Policy Fact Sheet, 16 November 1989, The White House, Office of the Press Secretary, plus attachment. In the area entitled "Force Application," the policy states that "The DOD will, consistent with treaty obligations, conduct research, development, and planning to be prepared to acquire and deploy space systems (for force application) should national security conditions dictate."

INDEX

THE AUTHOR

Simon P. Worden is a Colonel in the United States Air Force. Currently, he is Director for Advanced Concepts, Science and Technology, National Space Council, Executive Office of the President. He is a graduate of the National War College, National Defense University, where, as a Research Fellow, he also researched and wrote this study. Colonel Worden received a B.S. in physics and astronomy from the University of Michigan, and a Ph.D. in astronomy from the University of Arizona.

Colonel Worden's previous positions include the following: Chief of the Special Operations Branch, US Space Command; Senior Policy Analyst for the Office of Science and Technology Policy, Executive Office of the President; Special Assistant to the Director, Strategic Defense Initiative (SDI) Organization, Department of Defense, also serving as Advisor to the Delegation to the Negotiations on Nuclear and Space Arms with the Soviet Union; Executive Military Assistant to the Defensive Technologies Study (the technical basis for SDI); and Astrophysicist for the Air Force Geophysics Laboratory. Colonel Worden has twice received the Air Force Outstanding Research and Development Award for his work in astrophysics and optics.